Cell and Developmental Biology
of the Eye

Cell and Developmental Biology of the Eye

Series Editors
Joel B. Sheffield and S. Robert Hilfer

Ocular Size and Shape: Regulation During Development

Cellular Communication During Ocular Development

Molecular and Cellular Basis of Visual Acuity

The Proceedings of the Philadelphia Symposia on Ocular
and Visual Development

Molecular and Cellular Basis of Visual Acuity

Edited by
S. Robert Hilfer and
Joel B. Sheffield

With 72 Figures

Springer-Verlag
New York   Berlin   Heidelberg   Tokyo

S. Robert Hilfer
Joel B. Sheffield
Department of Biology
Temple University
Philadelphia, Pennsylvania 19122, U.S.A.

On the cover: Limulus photoreceptor turnover. See page 45.

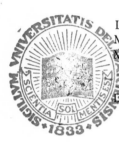

Library of Congress Cataloging in Publication Data
Main entry under title:
Molecular and cellular basis of visual acuity.
(Cell and developmental biology of the eye)
Papers from the Seventh Symposium on Ocular and Visual
Development, held in October 1982 in Philadelphia, Pa.
Bibliography: p.
Includes index.
1. Visual acuity—Congresses. 2. Retina—Congresses.
3. Photoreceptors—Congresses. I. Hilfer, S. Robert.
II. Sheffield, Joel B. III. Symposium on Ocular and
Visual Development (7th : 1982 : Philadelphia, Pa.)
IV. Series. [DNLM: 1. Visual acuity—Congresses.
W3 SY5363 7th 1982 / WW 145 M718] QP479.M65   1984
591.1'823   83-20436

Printed and bound by Halliday Lithograph Corporation,
West Hanover, Massachusetts
Printed in the United States of America.
9 8 7 6 5 4 3 2 1
ISBN 0-387-90964-8 Springer-Verlag New York Berlin Heidelberg Tokyo
ISBN 3-540-90964-8 Springer-Verlag Berlin Heidelberg New York Tokyo

Series Preface

The eye has fascinated scientists from the earliest days of biological investigation. The diversity of its parts and the precision of their interaction make it a favorite model system for a variety of developmental studies. The eye is a particularly valuable experimental system not only because its tissues provide examples of fundamental processes, but also because it is a prominent and easily accessible structure at very early embryonic ages.

In order to provide an open forum for investigators working on all aspects of ocular development, a series of symposia on ocular and visual development was initiated in 1973. A major objective of the symposia has been to foster communication between the basic research worker and the clinical community. It is our feeling that much can be learned on both sides from this interaction. The idea for an informal meeting allowing maximum exchange of ideas originated with Dr. Leon Canbeub, who supplied the necessary driving force that made the series a reality. Each symposium has concentrated on a different aspect of ocular development. Speakers have been selected to approach related topics from different perspectives.

This book series, "Cell and Developmental Biology of the Eye," is derived from the Philadelphia symposia on ocular and visual development. Previous volumes are listed on the series page. We hope that the introduction of this proceedings series will make the results of research on ocular cell and developmental biology more widely known and more easily accessible.

Preface

The Seventh Symposium on Ocular and Visual Development was held in October, 1982. The aim of the meeting was to develop a broad perspective on visual acuity. The subject was discussed initially in terms of molecular events of photoreception, and the metabolism of the photoreceptor elements. Subsequent papers presented the development and complexity of the neurocircuitry and transmitter systems in the retina that process the visual information prior to transfer to the brain. The meeting concluded with a series of papers on behavioral and physiological methods of measurement of visual acuity in humans, particularly young children. This volume arose from the papers presented at the meeting. We feel that the juxtaposition of research of broadly differing methodologies will be stimulating, rather than daunting, and will generate an enhanced understanding of this complex subject.

We are indebted to our colleagues: Dr. M. Mote from Temple University, and Drs. J. Siegfried, P. Dayhaw-Barker, and L. Press from the Pennsylvania College of Optometry for their expertise and assistance in the organization of the meeting; to the speakers for their presentations and contributions to this volume; and to the reviewers of the manuscripts for their helpful comments.

This symposium could not have been held without the generous support of the Temple University College of Arts and Sciences and the Pennsylvania College of Optometry. We also thank Merck, Sharp and Dohme, Inc. for their donation. This volume was prepared with the skills of Jo-Ann Felder and Michael Czeredarczuk. We thank them for their help.

October 23, 1983   S. Robert Hilfer
Philadelphia, Pennsylvania   Joel B. Sheffield

Contents

Contributors

J.P. Alligood, Laboratory of Vision Research, National Eye Institute, National Institutes of Health, Bethesda, MD 20205

R.B. Barlow, Institute for Sensory Research, Syracuse University, Syracuse, NY 13210

N.C. Brecha, Center for Ulcer Research and Education, Veterans Administration Medical Center, Wadsworth, Los Angeles, CA 90073 and Department of Medicine, Jules Stein Eye Institute, and Brain Research Institute, University of California at Los Angeles School of Medicine, Los Angeles, CA 90024

S.C. Chamberlain, Institue for Sensory Research, Syracuse University, Syracuse, NY 13210

V. Dobson, Department of Psychology, University of Washington, Seattle, WA 98195

P.A. Dudley, Laboratory of Vision Research, National Eye Institute, National Institutes of Health, Bethesda, MD 20205

H.J. Karten, Departments of Neurobiology and Behavior and Psychiatry and Behaviorial Sciences, SUNY at Stony Brook, Stony Brook, NY 11794

L. Kass, Institute for Sensory Research, Syracuse University, Syracuse, NY 13210

J-H. Kock, Department of Zoology, Division of Physiology, The University, Arkadian Katu 7, SF 00100 Helsinki 10, Finland

H. Kolb, Physiology Department, The University of Utah School of Medicine, Salt Lake City, UT 84108

P.A. Liebman, Department of Anatomy G3, The School of Medicine, University of Pennsylvania, Philadelphia, PA 19104

P.J. O'Brien, Laboratory of Vision Research, National Eye Institute, National Institutes of Health, Bethesda, MD 20205

L.A. Riggs, Walter S. Hunter Laboratory of Psychology, Brown University, Providence, RI 02912

S. Sokol, Department of Ophthalmology, Tufts University School of Medicine, New England Medical Center Hospital, 171 Harrison Avenue, Boston, MA 02111

W.K. Stell, Department of Anatomy, University of Calgary, Faculty of Medicine, 3330 Hospital Drive, N.W., Calgary, Alberta, Canada T2N 4N1

Control of Visual Receptor Cyclic GMP and Visual Excitation

P.A. Liebman

Psychophysical measurements have shown that human rods can detect single photons (Hecht et al, 1942). More recent electrophysiological recordings have demonstrated single photon responses (quantum bumps) in amphibian rods (Yau et al, 1977). These hyperpolarizing quantum bumps have a peak amplitude of about 1 millivolt or 1 picoampere and occur against a background of intrinsic rod electrical noise (Baylor et al, 1979). They are caused by a transient reduction in rod outer segment Na^+ conductance near the site of photon absorption. Quantum bumps follow photon absorption with a constant delay, amplitude and duration illustrated in Figure 1. The onset of conductance change has a characteristic shape mathematically equivalent to a process where a sequence of four consecutive first order chemicals intervenes between photon absorption and conductance change. Two of these four reactions are materially slower than the others (Baylor et al, 1980).

Photon absorption occurs on the rod disk membranes, physically separated from the rod outer segment plasma membrane. Thus, a cytoplasmic transmitter molecule probably carries the signal from the former to the later membrane where the Na^+ conductance is changed (Hagins, 1972). Finally, it is clear that if the transmitter is a common cellular constituent such as Ca^{++}, its concentration must be changed materially by the action of a single photon. This implies that tranduction must be mediated with considerable amplification. Analysis of the electrical dark noise of rod outer segments also shows that many Na^+ conductance channels must be controlled by a photon absorption, thus confirming the need for amplification (Schwartz, 1977).

In summary, to understand visual transduction, we must discover what biochemical mechanisms can account for sensitivity to a single photon, amplification (gain) of 1000 fold or more, and kinetics

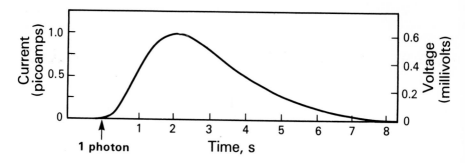

Figure 1.   Amplitude and time course of amphibian rod electrical response to a single photon (Sketch after Baylor et al., 1979).

(speed) characterized by a four stage formation process that finally decays as a single first-order process in about one second.   Though evidence has accumulated favoring the hypothesis that Ca^{++} is the amplified transmitter that blocks Na^+ conductance, there is as yet no detailed explanation for the kinetic nature of the delay or of the decay within the Ca^{++} hypothesis.   Recent work has revealed the presence of a set of light-activated enzymes that control cyclic GMP concentration in rod outer segments (Liebman & Pugh, 1981).   The sensitivity, amplification, and kinetics of activity buildup and decay of these enzymes come close to meeting all the requirements of the visual transduction mechanism.

METHOD

Retinas are removed from dark adapted eyes with the aid of infrared viewing devices.   Rod outer segments are separated from the retina by mechanical agitation (Vortex shaker), purified by buoyant density centrifugation and resuspended in physiologic salt solution containing 150 mM KCl, 2 mM $MgCl_2$, 2 mM DTT and 20 mM MOPS buffer. Aliquots of these rod disk membrane (RDM) suspensions containing 1 – 10 μM rhodopsin are assayed for cGMP phosphodiesterase (PDE) activity (after addition of cGMP and necessary cofactors) by a sensitive recording pH meter according to the method of Liebman and Evanczuk, (1981).   Thus, all experimental records seen in this paper show the production of protons vs. time caused by the reaction:

$$\text{cGMP} \underset{\text{PDE}}{\rightleftharpoons} 5' \text{ GMP}^- + \text{H}^+$$

Enzyme velocity is determined from the slope of the product curves (Figure 2). Slope or velocity in this work is proportional to number of active enzyme molecules in the presence of saturating substrate concentration. Buffering limits the pH change to about 0.1 unit per millimolar protons formed. A 1 msec duration xenon photoflash attentuated by calibrated neutral filters and a green wratten 57 filter is used for light activation. The fraction bleached is that determined from direct spectroscopic measurement of rhodopsin remaining after an unattentuated flash times the attentuation factor of the particular neutral filters used.

RESULTS

Figure 2 shows that in the presence of 100 µM GTP (necessary activation cofactor), light-activated cGMP hydrolysis is readily measured using the recording pH meter. Note that for the steepest curve activated by a large (15%) bleach, activity starts immediately after the light flash while the weaker activations occur only after a delay. The great light sensitivity of the preparation is clear

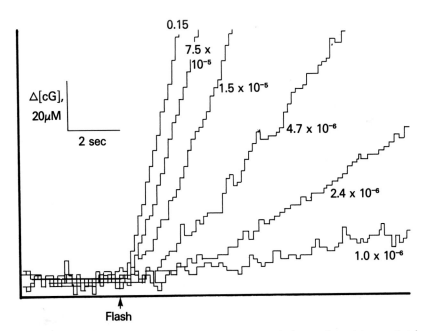

Figure 2. H^+ production (cGMP hydrolysis) as function of time after bleaching (arrow) fraction of rhodopsin labelling each curve. Toad RDM suspension (3 µM rhodopsin) in medium containing 8 mM cGMP and 500 µM GTP at 25°C. 1 msec flash (from Liebman & Pugh, 1981).

since the curve marked 1.5×10^{-4} bleach has nearly the same slope (velocity) as that for a 0.15 bleach. Figure 3 plots the maximum velocity achieved in each case against the fraction of rhodopsin bleached. The 63% semi-saturation of activation occurs with a bleach of 1/72,000 rhodopsins in toad and with a 1/10,000 to 1/25,000 rhodopsin bleach for cow RDM in the presence of GTP co-factor.

Examination of the 10^{-6} bleach curve of Figure 2 reveals a maximum velocity of about 3 μM cGMP/sec. in a preparation containing 3 μM rhodopsin, i.e., 1 mole cGMP/sec/mole rhodopsin content. But this velocity was caused by 10^{-6} mole bleached rhodopsin so that the specific activity was 1 mole cG/sec/10^{-6} mole bleached rhodopsin or 10^{6} cG/sec/R* (R* = activated or bleached rhodopsin). It would not be unreasonable to conclude that one R* molecule must have caused activation of one PDE molecule and each active PDE enzyme hydrolyzed (turned over) one million cGMP's each second, i.e., the turnover number of PDE is about $10^{6}s^{-1}$. However, we have shown from

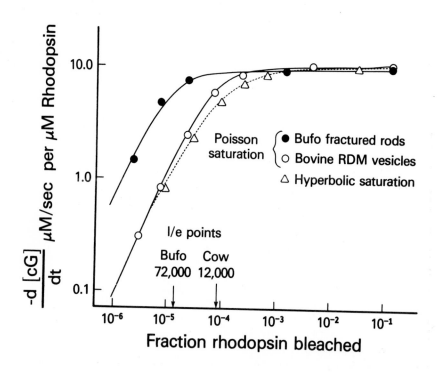

Figure 3. Light titration of maximum velocity of cGMP hydrolysis (-d[cGMP]/dt) determined from curves such as those of figure 2 for toad (Bufo marinus) and cow. Arrows indicate average fraction of rhodopsin bleached on a single disk to produce 63% of full activation.

basic considerations that PDE can not have a turnover number greater than about $10^4 s^{-1}$ and we were forced to conclude that some 100 or more PDE molecules were activated by each R* molecule formed by the bleach (Yee and Liebman, 1978; Liebman and Pugh, 1979)! Later work showed PDE to have a turnover number of 2000 s^{-1} (Baehr et al, 1982). Thus 500 PDE's are activated per R*, a 500 fold particle amplification.

A single R* could not activate 500 PDE's simultaneously, but it might do so sequentially. Such a process would have to proceed by a mechanism like sequential R*-PDE contact (Yee & Liebman, 1978; Liebman & Pugh, 1979). Since both R*-PDE and PDE are bound to the RDM membrane, 500 sequential contacts require diffusional mixing of these species on the membrane surface. The time required for such diffusional motion of rhodopsin had previously been measured by Liebman and Entine (1974) and others (Poo & Cone, 1974). A 63% completion time can be calculated by dividing the membrane surface area by the sum of the diffusion coefficients of the reactants. For a cow disk membrane, the calculated diffusional mixing time of 1 second compared well with the measured 1 second delay to 63% of full activity (Liebman & Pugh, 1979). Nevertheless, each newly contacted PDE would have to "remember" to stay active while subsequent R*-PDE contacts continued to build up and we hypothesized that this might explain the cofactor role of GTP in activation. R* might catalyze the opening of a GTP binding site on PDE. Each PDE·GTP complex would then remain active while the remaining PDE activations continued. If several R* were to be present within a single diffusional region or domain at higher bleaches, the PDE·GTP buildup in this domain would occur more quickly but the number of PDE's activated per domain would remain the same and the gain (PDE·GTP's per R*) would be less. At the same time, domains or disks previously unbleached at lower bleaches, would start to receive one or more photons at higher bleaches to produce higher net activity as the light titration curves show (Liebman & Pugh, 1979).

Subsequent to these early results, it was shown that R* causes GTP to bind not directly to PDE but to another protein that we call Γ (GTP-binding protein) (Godchaux & Zimmerman, 1979; Fung & Stryer, 1980). Γ is also bound to RDM (Goldchaux & Zimmerman, 1979) and we have found it present in about 6 fold molar excess over PDE (Sitaramaya & Liebman, MS in preparation). Thus, it seems that R* and Γ must initially interact diffusionally to yield Γ*·GTP's which then interact with PDE. Because of the excess over PDE, the theoretical membrane diffusional mixing time course for this mechanism of

PDE activity buildup could be identical to that previously attributed to direct R*-PDE interaction, the rate limiting step being Γ*·GTP activation.

It has been shown that each Γ is composed of three subunits, α, β, and γ (Fung, et al, 1980), the latter of which probably serves as a GTP'ase to remove the terminal phosphate group of the bound GTP molecule after several seconds (Shinozawa et al, 1980). The resulting GDP remains bound to Γ and is only displaced by another GTP that binds in exchange for GDP in the presence of R* (Fung & Stryer, 1980). Thus, it has been concluded that Γ's can continue to be activated, deactivated and reactivated in the presence of R* and GTP'ase.

Careful measurement of the number of GTP's bound per R* show amplification several-fold larger than the near simultaneous amplification of PDE's (Liebman & Pugh, 1982). Thus, the Γ·GTP to PDE coupling is de-amplified. For this reason, it appears that the Γ·GTP activator molecules are involved in a relatively weak steady-state binding interaction with the PDE (Sitaramayya & Liebman, MS in preparation). It is of profound significance for both Γ·GTP and PDE, that the amplification, light sensitivity and delay to maximum velocity are all greater with larger rod disk membrane area for toads and frogs (6 μm disk diameter) than for cows (1.5 μm disk diameter). This result is readily predicted by the diffusional-activation hypothesis.

Finally, by using the "non-hydrolyzable" GTP analogues, GMP-P(NH)P or GTP γS, it is easy to see that γ phosphate bond energy is not utilized to activate Γ (Liebman & Pugh, 1981; Yee & Liebman, 1978; Wheeler & Bitensky, 1977; Figure 4) and that, as expected, light sensitivity, amplification and delay to maximum velocity are increased together in the absence of GTP-hydrolytic deactivation in a predictable manner (Pugh & Liebman, 1980). Thus, R* appears to catalyze allosteric interaction between Γ and GTP, building up high populations of Γ·GTP until the rate of formation of new Γ·GTP's set by the diffusional mixing rate and size of the membrane is just equal to the rate of Γ·GTP loss due to GTP'ase action.

The figures illustrating the above discussed effects seem to show a relatively slow time course compared to the time course of the quantum bump response. However, when ATP is added to the other constituents, the activation of PDE appears and decays much more quickly (Liebman & Pugh, 1979; Liebman & Pugh, 1980; Figure 4). Previous work by Sitaramayya et al. (1977) showed that purified bleached rhodopsin could activate PDE but phosphorylated bleached rhodopsin could not. We have now shown in a number of ways that ATP works through rhodopsin-kinase-mediated multiple phosphorylation of R*. Thus, although GTP can be added even minutes after a light flash to produce activation, the prior introduction of ATP leaves GTP unable to activate Γ. If ATP is added at any time after light and GTP activation, the ongoing activity is promptly arrested or quenched. The speed of the quench with both GTP and ATP present is just slow enough to allow R* and GTP to activate the necessary few hundred PDE's before ATP-phosphorylation of R* inactivates it.

ATP analogues with non-transferable γ phosphate such as AMP P(CH$_2$)P or AMP P(NH)P cannot substitute for ATP. Instead, these analogues partially block the action of ATP (Liebman and Pugh, 1980). Small amounts of ATP (μM) produce parallel reduction of the Γ·GTP amplification and PDE amplification activated by R* suggesting that the lifetime of R* might be dramatically shortened by ATP (Liebman & Pugh, 1982). When Γ, PDE, and rhodopsin kinase are removed and purified from RDM, reconstitution of membranes containing only rhodopsin, Γ and PDE show amplified light-activation but ATP does not accelerate deactivation (quench). Addition of kinase allows ATP to quench the activation (Sitaramayya & Liebman, 1982).

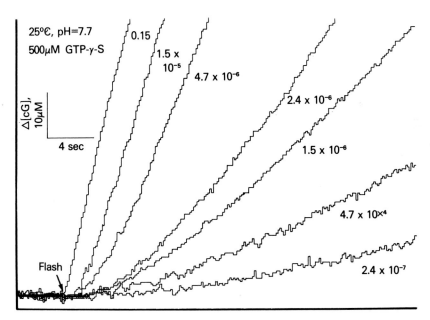

Figure 4.   Same experiment as figure 2 using GTP-γ-S instead of GTP. Curves show increased velocity per bleach with proportionally greater delay to maximum and increased light sensitivity as expected if binding of GTP but not hydrolysis were important for activation while GTP'ase reduces amplification helping to arrest activation.

8

Finally, we have shown that the time course of rhodopsin phosphorylation measured using γ-^{32}P-labelled ATP, is very fast, some 9–20 phosphates per R* being bound in about 1 second at weak bleaches. Figure 5 shows that the time course of PDE activation–deactivation in the presence of both GTP and ATP can be quite fast, the PDE velocity envelope being quite reminiscent of quantum bump shape and speed.

How might light-activated PDE activation control the reduction in Na^+ conductance that mediates visual transduction? Nichol & Miller (1978) have shown that direct injection of cGMP into rod outer segments depolarizes the cell membrane. Light activation shortens the duration of the cG-induced depolarization. In many cells whose function is activated by the water soluble hormones and in many cases of neurotransmitter action in the brain and spinal cord, the hormone or transmitter binding to a receptor protein at the cell membrane exterior surface causes GTP-binding to a protein activator of adenylate cyclase or of cyclic AMP (cAMP) phosphodiesterase at the membrane interior surface (Greengard, 1979). The activated enzyme changes the intracellular level of cAMP that in turn interacts with the regulatory subunit of a cAMP-dependent protein kinase. The active protein kinase uses ATP to phosphorylate yet another protein, an effector protein that then produces the

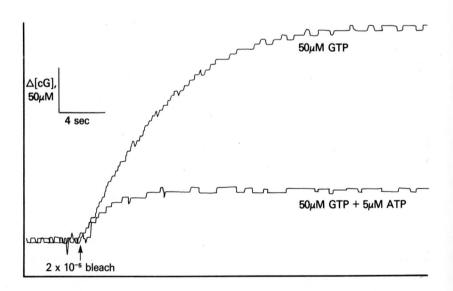

Figure 5a. Hydrolysis of cGMP after a weak bleach with GTP cofactor alone compared to reduced hydrolysis when ATP also present (from Liebman & Pugh, 1981).

physiologic final effect of the hormone or transmitter on the activated cell (Greengard, 1979). There is some evidence that cGMP similarly modulates the phosphorylation of proteins in rod outer segments (Polans et al, 1979).

Another possible physiologic effector produced by PDE activation might be H^+, the product of cGMP hydrolysis that we measure in our experiments above. Even with the reduced PDE amplification found in the presence of ATP in our experiments, 10^4 - 10^5 H^+ are produced per R* before the latter is incapacitated by phosphorylation.

What do these protons do? It is interesting that the amplified release of Ca^{++} that has recently been measured in intact retinas is also about 10^4 Ca^{++} per R* (Gold & Korenbrot, 1980; Yoshikami et al, 1980). Could the many H^+ produced by local cGMP hydrolysis cause the Ca^{++} to be released? Two such possible coupling mechanisms come to mind. First, Ca^{++} might be bound to cytoplasm constitutents and on disk membrane cytoplsmic surfaces to simple anionic sites. Both H^+ and Ca^{++} are small, intensely charged, freely diffusing ions that may compete for the same anionic binding sites. When the local H^+

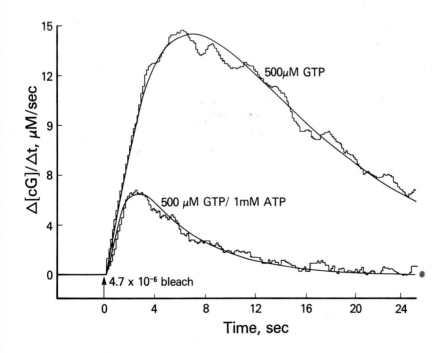

Figure 5b. Mathematical derivative of curves similar to those of 5a showing speed with which velocity ($\Delta[cG]/\Delta t$) develops and is quenched in the presence of ATP compared to that with GTP alone.

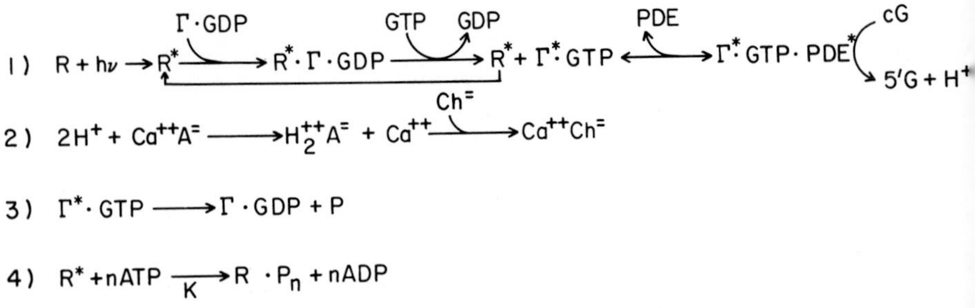

$$1)\quad R + h\nu \longrightarrow R^* \xrightarrow{\ \Gamma\cdot GDP\ } R^*\cdot\Gamma\cdot GDP \xrightarrow{\ GTP\quad GDP\ } R^* + \Gamma^*_*GTP \xleftrightarrow{\ PDE\ } \Gamma^*_*GTP\cdot PDE^*_* \nwarrow^{cG}_{\searrow 5'G + H^+}$$

$$2)\quad 2H^+ + Ca^{++}A^= \longrightarrow H_2^{++}A^= + Ca^{++} \xrightarrow{\ Ch^=\ } Ca^{++}Ch^=$$

$$3)\quad \Gamma^*\cdot GTP \longrightarrow \Gamma\cdot GDP + P$$

$$4)\quad R^* + nATP \xrightarrow[K]{} R\cdot P_n + nADP$$

Figure 6. Mechanism controlling cGMP in a rod and its possible effect on transduction. In reaction 1, light (hν) strikes rhodopsin, R, bleaching it to R* (metarhodopsin II). R* collides and sticks to Γ·GDP on the disk membrane surface forming R*·Γ·GDP which can exchange GDP for a GTP from the cytoplasm. R* is released to repeat this cycle with a new Γ·GDP while the Γ*·GTP formed can stick to a membrane PDE (Γ*·GTP·PDE*). This activated PDE complex hydrolyzes cGMP (cG) from the cytoplasm to generate 5'GMP and H$^+$. This mechanism activates several thousand Γ·GDP's and about 500 PDE's each second to yield about 10^6 H$^+$ after one second. Reaction 2 illustrates the hypothesized displacement of Ca^{++} from binding or storage sites, A$^=$, by H$^+$. Reactions 3 and 4 arrest the activated components. Γ*·GTP contains a GTP'ase that hydrolyzes bound GTP in about 2 seconds. R* is phosphorylated n times (n= 9 to 20) with the help of membrane bound rhodopsin kinase, K. This process is complete in under 1 second. The delayed but simultaneous activity of reactions 3 and 4 reduce the H$^+$ yield of reaction 1 to about 10^4–10^5 H$^+$ per R*.

suddenly rises, many of the bound Ca^{++} might be forced off their local sites, to diffuse away to the cell membrane and bind to the Na$^+$ channels to close them. Alternatively, the liberated H$^+$ may provide the energy for an H$^+$/Ca^{++} exchange pump on the disk membrane that permits Ca^{++} to escape from the disk interiors as the H$^+$ enters.

A model that summarizes the results and discussion above is shown in Figure 6. Clearly, many important tests of these ideas remain to be done.

Research of this laboratory is supported by NEI Grants EY00012 and EY01583.

REFERENCES

Baehr, W., Morita, E.A., Swanson, R.H. and Applebury, M.L. (1982) Characterization of bovine outer segment G-protein. J. Biol. Chem. 257: 6452-6460.

Baylor, D.A., Lamb, T.D. and Yau, K.-W. (1979) Responses of retinal rods to single photons. J. Physiol. 288: 613-634.

Baylor, D.A., Matthews, G. and Yau, K.-W. (1980) Two components of electrical dark noise in toad rod outer segments. J. Physiol. 309: 591-621.

Fung, B.K.-K., Hurley, J.B. and Stryer, L. (1981) Flow of information in the light-triggered cyclic nucleotide cascade of vision. Proc. Natl. Acad. Sci. U.S.A. 78: 152-156.

Fung, B.K.-K. and Stryer, L. (1980) Photolyzed rhodopsin catalyzes the exchange of GTP for bound GDP in retinal rod outer segments. Proc. Natl. Acad. Sci. U.S.A. 77: 2500-2504.

Godchaux, W. and Zimmerman, W.F. (1979) Membrane-dependent guanine nucleotide binding and GTPase activities of soluble protein from bovine rod cell outer segments. J. Biol. Chem. 254: 7874-7884.

Gold, G.H. and Korenbrot, J.I. (1980) Light induced calcium release by intact retinal rods. Proc. Natl. Acad. Sci. U.S.A. 77: 5557-5561.

Greengard, P. (1979) Some chemical aspects of neurotransmitter action. Trends. Pharm. Sci. 1: 27-29.

Hagins, W.A. (1972) The visual process: Excitatory mechanisms in the primary receptor cells. Ann. Revs. Biophys. Bioeng. 1: 131-158.

Hecht, S., Schlaer, S. and Pirenne, M. (1942) Energy, quanta & vision. J. Gen. Physiol. 25: 819-840.

Liebman, P.A. and Entine, G. (1974) Lateral diffusion of visual pigment in photoreceptor disk membranes. Science 185: 457-459.

Liebman, P.A. and Evanczuk, A.T. (1981) Real time assay of rod disk membrane cGMP phosphodiesterase and its controller enzymes. Meth. in Enzymol. 81: 532-542.

Liebman, P.A. and Pugh, E.N., Jr. (1979) The control of phosphodiesterase in rod disk membranes: Kinetics, possible mechanisms, and significance for vision. Vision Res. 19: 375-380.

Liebman, P.A. and Pugh, E.N., Jr. (1980) ATP mediates rapid reversal of cyclic GMP phosphodiesterase activation in visual receptor membranes. Nature 287: 734-736.

Liebman, P.A. and Pugh, E.N., Jr. (1981) Control of rod disk membrane phosphodiesterase and a model for visual transduction. Current Topics in Membrane Transport 15: 157-170.

Liebman, P.A. and Pugh, E.N., Jr. (1982) Gain, speed and sensitivity of GTP binding versus PDE activation in visual excitation. Vis. Res. 22: 1475-1480.

Nichol, G.D. and Miller, W.H. (1978) Cyclic GMP injected into retinal rod outer segments increases latency and amplitude of response to illumination, Proc. Natl. Acad. Sci. U.S.A. 75: 5217-5220.

Polans, A.S., Hermolin, J. and Bownds, M.D. (1979) Light-induced dephosphorylation of two proteins in frog rod outer segments. J. Gen. Physiol. 74: 595-613.

Poo, M.-M. and Cone, R. (1974) Lateral diffusion of rhodopsin in the photoreceptor membrane. Nature 247: 438-441.

Pugh, E.N., Jr. and Liebman, P.A. (1980) Delays and sensitivity support the lateral diffusion hypothesis of multiple PDE activation by single rhodopsin. Biophysical Journal 29: Abstracts of the Annual Meeting.

Schwartz, E.A. (1977) Voltage noise observed in rods of the turtle retina. J. Physiol. 272: 217-246.

Shinozawa, T., Uchida, S., Martin, E., Cafiso, D., Hubbell, D. and Bitensky, M.W. (1980) Additional component required for activity and reconstitution of light-activated vertebrate photoreceptor GTPase. Proc. Natl. Acad. Sci. U.S.A. 77: 1408-1411.

Sitaramayya, A. and Liebman, P.A. (1982) Mechanism of ATP quench of PDE activation in rod disk membranes. J. Biol. Chem. 258: 1205-1209.

Sitaramayya, A., Virmaux, N. and Mandel, P. (1977) On a soluble system for studying light activation of rod outer segment cyclic GMP phosphodiesterase. Neurochem. Res. 2: 1-10.

Wheeler, G.L. and Bitensky, M.W. (1977) A light-activated GTPase in vertebrate photoreceptors: Regulation of light-activated cyclic GMP phosphodiesterase. Proc. Natl. Acad. Sci. U.S.A. 74: 4238-4242.

Yau, K.-W., Lamb, T.D. and Baylor, D.A. (1977) Light-induced fluctuations in membrane current of single toad rod outer segments. Nature 269: 78-80.

Yee, R. and Liebman, P.A. (1978) Light-activated phosphodiesterase of the rod outer segment. J. Biol. Chem. 253: 8902-8909.

Yoshikami, S., George, J.S. and Hagins, W.A. (1980) Light-induced calcium fluxes from the outer segment layer of vertebrate retinas. Nature 286: 395-398.

Biochemical Events Related to Circadian Photoreceptor Shedding

P.A. Dudley, J.P. Alligood and P.J. O'Brien

The renewal of vertebrate photoreceptor outer segments is accomplished by the assembly of new disc membranes at the base and
shedding of old membranes at the distal tip of the outer segment
(Young and Bok, 1969). This intermittent shedding process occurs
shortly after the onset of light in animals entrained to a schedule
of 12 hours of light and 12 hours of darkness and follows a circadian rhythm in rats (LaVail, 1976, 1980; Goldman et al, 1980) but
is light-driven in frogs (Basinger et al., 1976; Hollyfield et al,
1976). In Xenopus laevis, both circadian and light-driven
mechanisms can be expressed depending on experimental conditions
(Besharse et al, 1977a). The immediate regulation of light-driven
shedding in the frog resides in the eye itself (Hollyfield and
Basinger, 1978). The same is true of circadian shedding in the rat,
with the added complication that re-entrainment of the retinal
pacemaker requires input from the central nervous system (Teirstein,
Goldman and O'Brien, 1980). These processes have been reviewed
recently by Besharse (1982).

In both frogs and Xenopus the onset of light initiates not only
shedding of the tip but also accelerated membrane renewal at the
base of the outer segment (Besharse et al. 1977b). As a result, the
membrane lost in the shedding response is replaced during the subsequent daylight hours. This rapid assembly of new membranes is not
a reflection of a transient stimulation of synthesis of the membrane
components since there is only a light elevation of opsin synthesis
in the frog (Matsumo and Bok, 1979) and no elevation detectable in
the synthesis of either opsin or total protein in Xenopus (Hollyfield et al, 1982). No morphological study has been carried out
with rat retinas to determine whether there might be a comparable
accelerated membrane assembly after shedding. However, preliminary
studies have shown elevated phospholipid synthesis during the day-

light hours (Dudley and O'Brien, 1981). Consequently a search was made for biochemical correlates to circadian photoreceptor shedding with emphasis on the major components of the outer segment disc membranes: opsin and phospholipids.

METHODS

Sprague-Dawley rats, 125-150g, from Zivic Miller Laboratories, Inc., Allison Park, PA, were maintained on a strict light cycle from birth, with the lights coming on at 7 A.M. and going off at 7 P.M. Light levels within the cages never exceeded 10-20 foot-candles. For experiments involving constant light or constant darkness the lights were turned on or off at the usual time but were prevented from cycling further. At various times animals were sacrificed by exposure to carbon dioxide gas, under the prevailing light conditions, the eyes were enucleated, and the retinas were rapidly dissected out and placed in 5 ml RPMI 1640 medium (Gibco) supplemented with penicillin, 35 units per ml, streptomycin, 35 µg per ml, and HEPES buffer (N-2-hydroxyethyl-piperazine-N-2-ethane sulfonic acid) 30 mM, pH 7.4. For protein synthesis studies, leucine was omitted from the medium and one retina was incubated in each flask for 1.5 hr with 50 µCi $1-(4,5^3H)$-leucine (52.2 to 56.5 Ci/mmole). For glycoprotein synthesis studies the glucose content of the medium was reduced from 11 mM to 1.1 mM and 1 mM pyruvate was added. Single retinas were then incubated with 50 µCi of either D-$(1,6-^3H)$-glucosamine hydrochloride (39.6 Ci/mmole) for 1.5 hr or D-$(1-^3H)$-galactose (14.2 Ci/mmole) for 2 hr. For lipid synthesis studies 2 retinas were incubated in each flask for 45 min with 50 uCi of $(2-^3H)$ glycerol (10 Ci/mmole). All isotopes were from New England Nuclear. Incubations were carried out at 37^oC in a shaking water bath with a 0.1 liter/min flow of 95% oxygen/5% CO_2 in each flask. Incubations were run in triplicate for lipids and in quadruplicate for proteins and glycoproteins. Retinas were collected by centrifugation and washed with phosphate-buffered saline (PBS).

Crude ROS were prepared by suspending 2 retinas in 1 ml 34 percent (w/v) sucrose in 65 mM NaCl containing 2 mM $MgCl_2$ and 5 mM tris-acetate, pH 7.4. ROS were broken off with ten 3 sec bursts of a vortex mixer. After 10 minutes of centrifugation at 15,000 xg the floating ROS were removed from the retinal debris, which was resuspended in another 1 ml sucrose solution. The procedure was repeated and the combined ROS suspensions were diluted with 6 ml PBS for centrifugation at 27,000 xg for 10 minutes.

Lipids were extracted with chloroform-methanol (2:1, v/v) and the extract was washed by the method of Folch et al., (1957). The chloroform layer was evaporated to dryness under N_2 and the lipids were re-solubilized in chloroform for two dimensional thin layer chromatography on silica gel H plates (Analtec, Newark, DE) by the method of Anderson et al, (1970). After visualizing the phospholipids with iodine vapors, the spots were scaped off the plate and extracted with Bligh and Dyer (1959) monophase. Aliquots were taken for scintillation counting and for phosphorus determination (Rouser et al, 1966).

For electrophoretic separation of labeled opsin the incubated retinas were washed twice in PBS by centrifugation for 15 minutes at 27,000 xg. Each retina was suspended in 2 ml of 4 mM tris-acetate buffer, pH 7.4, containing 0.2 mM EDTA and 2% mercaptoethanol and sonicated with 3 bursts of about 5 seconds each using setting 3 of a Branson sonifer. The membrane fraction was sedimented by centrifugation for 30 minutes at 48,000 xg. The pellet was suspended in 225 µl tris-acetate-EDTA-mercaptoethanaol to which was added 25 µl 25% sodium dodecyl sulfate (SDS) in the same buffer. After 12 hr at room temperature 50 µl aliquots of the solubilized proteins were subjected to precipitation with 1 ml ethanol-ether (2:1,v/v). Pellets were collected by centrifugation and dissolved in 0.5 ml 1N NaOH with heating. Aliquots were taken for scintillation counting and protein determination by the method of Lowry et al, (1951). Aliquots of the SDS-extracts were diluted with an equal volume of 50% glycerol containing 0.002% bromphenol blue for electrophoresis on 7.5% polyacrylamide gels by the method of Fairbanks et al. (1971). Duplicate gels were run and one was stained with Coomassie Brilliant Blue. The other was cut into 1 mm slices which were placed in scintillation vials and digested overnight at 50° in NCS solubilizer (Amersham) containing 10% H_2O. Counting was done in a toluene-based scintillation fluid. Tissues were processed for light microscope autoradiography by the acetone dehydration method of Gould and Dawson (1976) as modified by Anderson and Hollyfield (1981).

RESULTS

The synthesis of rat retinal membrane proteins was examined by in vitro incubation of retinas with (^{3}H) leucine. Animals were enucleated at various times during the diurnal light-dark cycle. The retinas were incubated and membrane proteins were prepared as described in Methods. Measurement of the specific activity showed (figure 1) that there was very little variation in the rate of membrane protein synthesis throughout the 24 hour cycle, exhibiting only a slight elevation just prior to light onset. The rate of leucine incorporation was linear for at least two hours under these conditions and was not affected by light. Incorporation at 10 A.M. amounted to 1159 $\pm$ 394 DPM/µg protein (n=4) in 1.5 hours for retinas from animals maintained in darkness, compared with 1272 $\pm$ 344 DPM/µg protein (n=4) for retinas from animals that experienced the normal 7 A.M. onset of light.

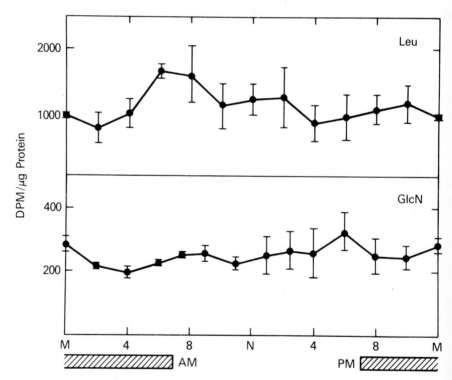

Figure 1. Specific activity of rat retina membrane proteins as a function of the lighting cycle. Rat retinas isolated at the indicated times were incubated with either (^{3}H) leucine (Leu) or (^{3}H) glucosamine (GlcN) and the membrane fraction was prepared and analyzed as described in Methods. Disintegrations/min (DPM)/µg protein are plotted against clock hours with the shaded area representing the period of darkness.

Membrane glycoprotein synthesis was monitored by in vitro incubation of retinas with (^{3}H) glucosamine. Because glucosamine is derived from glucose, the medium has to be altered to minimize dilution of the radioactive precursor while maintaining optimal protein synthesis. Table I shows that lowering the glucose content of the medium increased the incorporation of labeled glucosamine but that elimination of glucose was detrimental. However, supplementation with pyruvate restored acceptable levels of incorporation and maintained protein synthesis at the same level found with the full complement of glucose. Under these conditions incorporation was linear up to two hours with no effect of light detectable and with no diurnal variation (figure 1).

In order to determine if photoreceptor outer segment membrane synthesis was specifically undergoing a diurnal rhythm that was masked by the other retinal membrane proteins, the membrane proteins were solubilized in SDS and subjected to gel electrophoresis. A typical radioactive pattern of (^{3}H) glucosamine-labeled proteins is shown in figure 2. A similar pattern is produced with (^{3}H) leucine labeling. The major radioactive peak has been shown (Battelle and LaVail, 1980) to be opsin and is highly labeled by both precursors. It lags behind the major Coomassie Blue-staining band on the gels because the newly-synthesized opsin has an oligosaccharide chain that is subsequently shortened (Liang et al., 1979). If outer segment membrane synthesis were to vary throughout the day it should be reflected as a variation in opsin labeling relative to the general background of retinal membrane protein labeling. Figure 3 shows that the label in opsin was a constant percentage of the label in all the other higher molecular weight proteins on the gel. Neither (^{3}H) leucine nor (^{3}H) glucosamine labeling of opsin give any evidence of diurnal variation. Consequently, both the synthesis of the opsin polypeptide and its subsequent core glycosylation appear

TABLE I

EFFECT OF GLUCOSE CONCENTRATION ON GLUCOSAMINE INCORPORATION

	DPM/µg protein	
Carbon Source in Medium	(^{3}H) Glucosamine	(^{3}H) Leucine
Glucose 11 mM	22 $\pm$ 4	1,412 $\pm$ 246
Glucose 3.3 mM	46 $\pm$ 7	
Glucose 1.1 mM	85 $\pm$ 51	
None	56 $\pm$ 10	
Glucose 1.1 mM + pyruvate 1 mM	107 $\pm$ 11	1,478 $\pm$ 15

Rat retinas were incubated with (^{3}H) glucosamine or (^{3}H) leucine and the membrane fraction was prepared and analyzed as described in Methods.

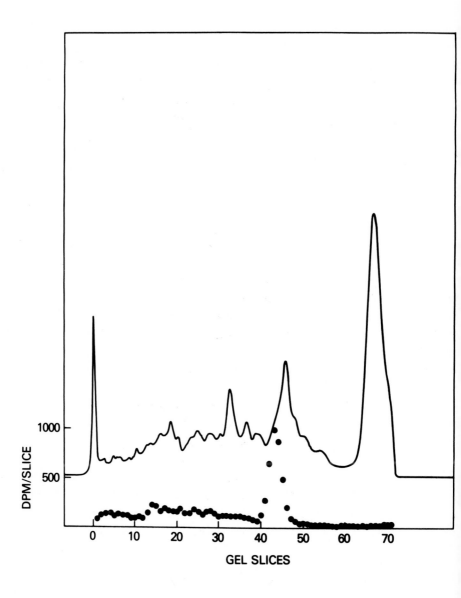

Figure 2. Distribution of labeled membrane proteins on SDS poly-acrylamide gels. Rat retinas were incubated with (^{3}H) glucosamine and the membrane fraction prepared for SDS gel electrophoresis as described in Methods. The Coomassie blue-stained gel is shown at the top of the figure. A densitometric scan of that gel is plotted as a solid line and the disintegrations/min (DPM) in each gel slice are shown in the dotted line.

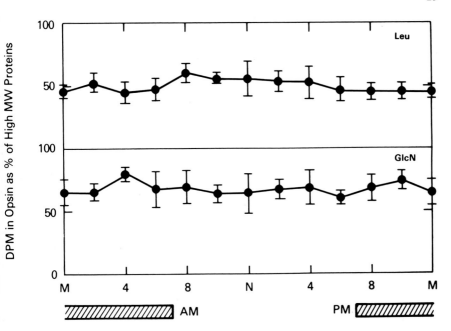

Figure 3. Radioactivity in opsin relative to other retinal membrane proteins as a function of the lighting cycle. Rat retinas were incubated at the indicated times with either (^{3}H) leucine (Leu) or (^{3}H) glucosamine (GlcN). The membrane fractions were prepared and solubilized for SDS gel electrophoresis as described in Methods. The disintegrations/min (DPM) in the opsin peaks were compared to the remaining higher molecular weight proteins on the gels. Those ratios expressed as percent are plotted for each precursor against clock hours. The shaded area represents the period of darkness.

to occur at a constant rate throughout the diurnal light cycle.

The incorporation of (^{3}H) galactose into opsin was used as a possible measure of the intracellular transport of opsin from cis- to trans-Golgi compartments (Bergeron et al, 1982). Because galactose is readily incorporated into glycogen in the retina (O'Brien and Muellenberg, 1968) the labeling of the entire membrane fraction was not measured. Crude rod outer segments were prepared and figure 4 shows a relatively constant level of galactose labeling of ROS with a slight elevation shortly after light offset. The labeling of opsin relative to the other glycoproteins in the crude ROS preparation showed a similar pattern. The elevation in ROS labeling at 8 P.M. thus represents, for the most part, a minor elevation in opsin labeling.

For studies of phospholipid synthesis, retinas were incubated with (^{3}H) glycerol to introduce label into all classes of phospholipids. For analysis the retinas were divided into a crude ROS fraction and retinal debris as described in Methods. After extrac-

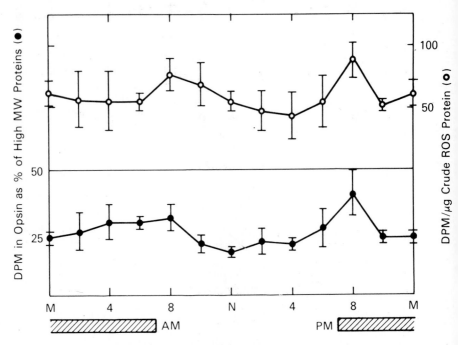

Figure 4. Incorporation of galactose into crude outer segment (ROS) proteins and opsin as a function of the lighting cycle. Rat retinas were incubated at the indicated times with (^{3}H) galactose. The ROS were prepared and solubilized for SDS gel electrophoresis as described in Methods. The upper curve shows distintegrations/min (DPM)/µg crude ROS protein (O) and the lower curve DPM in opsin as a percent of the DPM in higher molecular weight proteins on the gels (●). The abscissa is clock hours with the shaded area representing the period of darkness.

tion and two-dimensional thin layer chromatography (TLC), the specific activity was determined for three major phospholipid components: phosphatidylcholine (PC), phosphatidylethanolamine (PE) and phosphatidylinositol (PI). Phosphatidylserine was not measured because of the generally low specific activity.

It can be seen in figures 5-7 that in ROS, all three phospholipids exhibited elevated synthesis during the day with a sharp drop to markedly lower levels at light offset. The rate of synthesis remained low throughout the night and rose again at the onset of light. Phosphatidylinositol exhibited the greatest differential between day and night labeling of ROS phospholipids. The debris remaining after isolation of ROS was also extracted and the phospho-

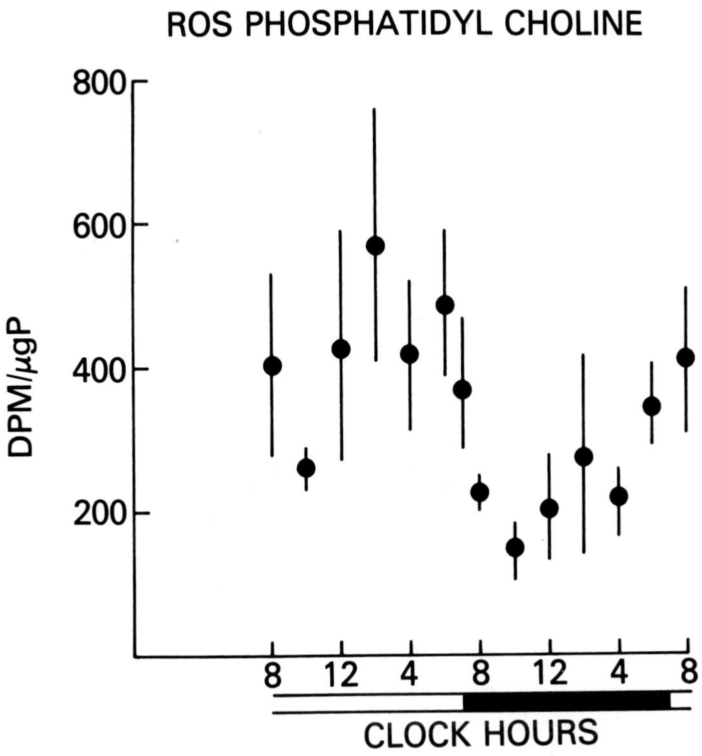

ROS PHOSPHATIDYL CHOLINE

Figure 5. Specific activity of rod outer segment (ROS) phosphatidylcholine as a function of the light cycle. Rat retinas were incubated at the indicated times with (^{3}H) glycerol. ROS were prepared and the phospholipids separated as described in Methods. Disintegrations/min (DPM)/µg phosphorus (P) are plotted against clock hours. The error lines around each point represent the standard deviation of the determinations. The shaded area represents the period of darkness.

lipids were chromatographed as before. Table II shows that there was a significant difference between the daytime and night time labeling of all three phospholipids not only in the ROS but also in the retinal debris. However, the debris contained some ROS which could influence the results. The ROS preparation was designed to yield as pure a sample as could be expected with a one-step procedure since the experiments required a large number of preparations. Consequently the sucrose concentration was kept low to minimize contaminants but with a lowered yield of ROS membranes.

In order to determine if the diurnal rhythms in phospholipid synthesis were governed by a ciracadian pacemaker some animals were maintained for one day in darkness and their retinal phospholipid synthesis measured as before. At the same time, other animals were

ROS PHOSPHATIDYL ETHANOLAMINE

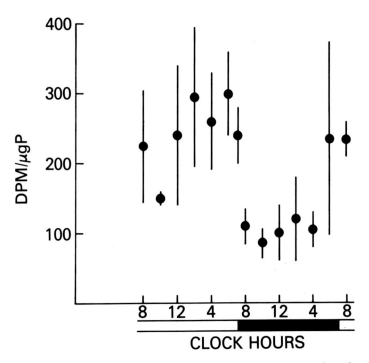

Figure 6. Specific activity of rod outer segment (ROS) phosphatidylethanolamine as a function of the lighting cycle. See legend to figure 5.

maintained in constant light to determine whether the elevated synthesis was a direct result of illumination. Both groups were compared with animals maintained on the normal cyclic light schedule. Table III shows that ROS PI synthesis was elevated in animals maintained in darkness at 3 P.M. when compared with control animals at 10 P.M. This effect suggested that the diurnal rhythm was in fact circadian. In addition to a circadian rhythm, PI also exhibited a light-stimulated elevation in labeling in the ROS. A similar light stimulation was evident in the retinal debris at 10 P.M. The specific activity of PI in the debris was 29,447 $\pm$ 4460 (n=4) DPM/µg P in the dark. This value rose to 75,238 $\pm$ 9837 (n=4) DPM/µg P in constant light. For comparison, the value found at 3 P.M. in the light was 71,136 $\pm$ 11,312 (n=4) DPM/µg P. Analysis of seven different experiments revealed (table IV) that only at night was there a significant stimulation of synthesis by light and only PI exhibited this effect which was seen in both ROS and retinal debris.

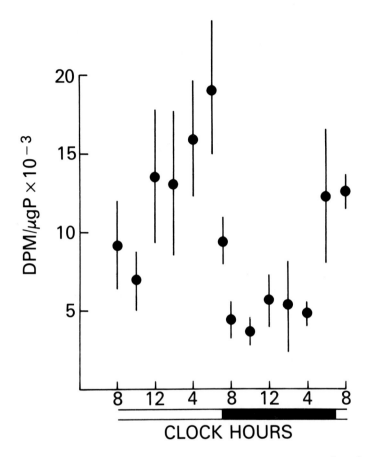

Figure 7. Specific activity of rod outer segment (ROS) phosphatidylinositol as a function of the lighting cycle. See legend to
figure 5.

The circadian nature of the diurnal rhythms in phospholipid
synthesis was demonstrated by maintaining animals in constant
darkness for three days before measuring (^{3}H) glycerol incorporation
at 2:30 P.M. and at 10 P.M. Table V shows that all three phospholipids exhibited significant differences between 2:30 and 10 P.M.
labeling in the ROS. Both PC and PE also exhibited significant
differences in the retinal debris but PI showed only a marginally
significant difference.

Previous work (Teirstien, et al., 1980) had shown that the
circadian pacemaker controlling photoreceptor shedding cycles was
located in the eye. Presumably the same pacemaker might govern the
phospholipid cycles. However, control of the light stimulation of
PI synthesis could be mediated by agents external to the eye. In

TABLE II
DIURNAL VARIATION IN PHOSPHOLIPID SYNTHESIS

| | DPM/µg phosphorus | | |
	PC	PE	PI
Crude ROS			
Day (n=9)	523 + 160	310 + 77	17,859 + 4,687
Night (n=8)	189 + 61	97 + 27	4,529 + 1,623
	p<0.001	p<0.001	p<0.001
Retinal Debris			
Day (n=9)	1,746 + 322	1,369 + 317	33,877 + 8,318
Night (n=8)	1,012 + 282	648 + 272	12,167 + 3,529
	p<0.001	p<0.001	p<0.001

Retinas were incubated with (^{3}H) glycerol and fractionated and the phospholipids were separated as described in Methods. Day = 2,4 and 6 PM; Night = 8 and 10 PM and 12 M.

PC = phosphatidylcholine; PE = phosphatidylethanolamine
PI = phosphatidylinositol; ROS = rod outer segments

order to resolve this question, retinas from animals maintained in darkness were incubated either in darkness or in the light. The specific activity of PI in the light was 26,490 $\pm$ 721 DPM/µg phosphorus and in darkness it was 13,365 $\pm$ 2,383 DPM/µg phosphorus (n=2; p<0.025). Thus light was capable of elevating the rate of PI synthesis in vitro and the control mechanism must reside in the retina.

In searching for biochemical events related to photoreceptor shedding, ROS were examined apart from the remainder of the retina. However, since the labeling time with (^{3}H) glycerol was only 45 min it did not seem likely that extensive labeling of the ROS could take place. Nevertheless, the ROS fraction was highly radioactive. Accordingly, an autoradiographic study was undertaken to determine the site of photoreceptor labeling. Figure 8 is a light microsopic autoradiogram of a rat retina incubated with (^{3}H) glycerol for 45 min in the light at 10 P.M. The pattern of labeling was essentially the same regardless of the time of day or the light conditions. It

TABLE III
EFFECT OF AMBIENT LIGHTING ON ROS PHOSPHATIDYLINOSITOL SYNTHESIS

Lighting Conditions	DPM/µg P	
	3 PM	10 PM
Cyclic light (on 7 AM off 7 PM)	28,688 + 5,077	3,656 + 861
Constant light	—	23,191 + 10,354
Constant darkness	18,603 + 2,599	—

Animals were maintained on the indicated lighting conditions and retinas were incubated with (^{3}H) glycerol under the same conditions. Fractionation and phospholipid separation was as described in Methods.

TABLE IV
LIGHT STIMULATION OF PHOSPHOLIPID SYNTHESIS
DURING THE DAY OR NIGHT

Significance Levels (p)
of Difference of Means

	PC	PE	PI
Crude ROS			
Day (n=20)	>0.2	>0.7	>0.1
Night (n=30)	>0.7	>0.7	<0.01
Retinal Debris			
Day (n=24)	>0.4	>0.4	>0.5
Night (n=32)	>0.4	>0.5	<0.001

Retinas were taken during the day (12-4 PM) or at night (9-10 PM) from each of two groups of animals maintained either in darkness or in the light. The retinas were then incubated with (^{3}H) glycerol as described in Methods under the same conditions of darkness or light. The mean values from 7 pooled experiments were subjected to a Student's t test where n is the number of determinations evenly divided between darkness and light. Abbreviations as in Table II.

should be noted that the differences in the summed radioactivity of all the phospholipids shown in table II amounted to an increase of 227 percent in the ROS and 215 percent in the retinal debris when comparing the daytime values with the night values. Relatively small differences such as these might not be expected to be apparent when using a technique such as autoradiography.

The greatest concentration of radiactivity occured in the rod inner segments. In contrast, there was very little label to be found in the ROS. The perinuclear region and both inner and outer synaptic layers were heavily labeled. The label in the ROS was a very small fraction of the total label throughout the retina. In parallel experiments, retinas were incubated and ROS were prepared as described in Methods. The phospholipid containing chloroform-

TABLE V
CIRCADIAN PHOSPHOLIPID SYNTHESIS AFTER 3 DAYS OF DARKNESS

	PC	DPM/µg phosphorus PE	PI
Crude ROS			
2:30 PM (n=4)	882 + 282	640 + 191	15,050 + 5,063
10:00 PM (n=4)	393 + 100	255 + 33	6,200 + 693
	p<0.025	p<0.01	p<0.025
Retinal Debris			
2:30 PM (n=4)	1,673 + 332	1,400 + 170	25,600 + 7,465
10:00 PM (n=4)	975 + 160	665 + 84	15,725 + 3,420
	p<0.01	p<0.001	p>0.05

Retinas were incubated with (^{3}H) glycerol and fractionated and the phospholipids were separated as described in Methods. Abbreviations as in Table II.

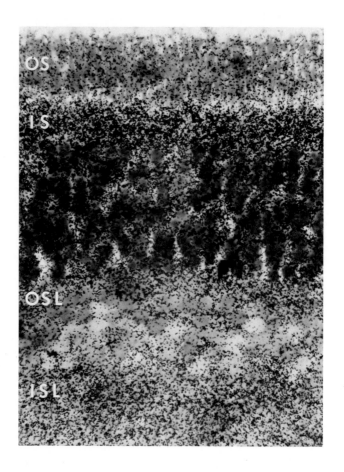

Figure 8. Light microscopic autoradiography of a rat retina incubated with (^{3}H) glycerol at 10 PM in the light. Incubation and tissue preparation is as described in Methods. Rod outer segments (OS) are lightly labeled whereas the inner segments (IS) are intensely labeled. The perinuclear region of the photoreceptors and the outer synaptic layer (OSL) as well as the inner synaptic layer (ISL) are also heavily labeled. Exposure time was 6 weeks.

methanol extracts of both ROS and retina debris were absorbed on silica gel, eluted with chloroform-methanol and the radioactivity was determined. Quadruplicate samples of 4 retinas each gave a distribution of 13,713 ± 2,129 DPM in ROS and 64,701 ± 25,854 DPM in retinal debris. Although 17.5 percent of the radioactivity was in the ROS fraction, the autoradiogram suggested a much smaller fraction.

In another parallel experiment quadruplicate samples of 4 retinas each were incubated and a membrane fraction was prepared and dehydrated as described in Methods. Subsequent extraction with chloroform-methanol yielded 71,178 ± 11,439 DPM which agreed closely with the sum of the ROS and retinal debris extracts, i.e., 78,414 DPM. However, the residue remaining after chloroform-methanol extraction still contained 95,028 ± 25,739 DPM, probably in glycogen and protein (Bibb and Young, 1974; Mercurio and Holtzman, 1982b). Thus, only 43 percent of the incorporated label was in phospholipid, reducing the ROS fraction to 7.5 percent of the total in the retina. Since ROS represent about 10 percent of the retina, this amount of label would require a uniform distribution of radioactivity across the entire retina. The autoradiogram shows that this was not the case. Consequently, the ROS fractions must contain membranes derived from the inner segment, probably with similar lipid composition and density.

DISCUSSION

The circadian rhythm in phospholipid synthesis is not a reflection of a general metabolic rhythm since protein synthesis does not fluctuate significantly. Furthermore, it probably does not reflect a change in the endogeneous pools of phospholipid precursors since light stimultion of PI synthesis at night produces specific activities comparable to those seen in the daylight hours in both ROS and retinal debris. This would not be possible if the unlabeled endogenous pools were larger during the night. Consequently, the rhythm appears to reflect actual fluctuations in the amounts of phospholipids synthesized.

The existence of a circadian rhythm in the synthesis of ROS phospholipid provides a biochemical basis for the earlier observation (Goldman, et al., 1980) that photoreceptor outer segment shedding could not be induced in rat retinas until approximately 24 hours had elapsed since the previous shedding event. The elevated synthesis of the phospholipids occurs during the day and would appear to provide sufficient membrane to replace any that might be shed during the remainder of the 24 hour cycle. However, the synthesis of opsin, the major ROS membrane protein, exhibits no such rhythmicity. Rather, opsin is synthesized at a constant rate at all times. As a consequence, initially the rapidly synthesized membranes would be quite low in their opsin/phospholipid ratio. This ratio would increase with time as additional opsin molecules were inserted into the membranes, ultimately reaching the value requisite for ROS disc membrane assembly. The fact that shedding in the rat cannot be induced more frequently than once every day suggests that

rat photoreceptors may regulate shedding by monitoring the composition of the precursor membranes.

Opsin synthesis in Xenopus laevis, the clawed frog, likewise
exhibits no diurnal fluctuation (Hollyfield, et al., 1982) even
though new disc membrane assembly occurs during the first 8 hours of
light exposure (Besharse, et al, 1977b). Other similarities exist
between rat and Xenopus in that the latter is capable of exhibiting
a latent circadian rhythm of shedding (Besharse, et al, 1977a).
Furthermore, Papermaster et al (1979) found opsin-containing vesicles in the inner segment of Xenopus rods near the base of the
connecting cilium and Papermaster and Schneider (1982) reported
opsin in membrane cisternae located parallel to the ciliary rootlet
in rat rods. Thus, in both animals there appears to be a pool of
pre-formed opsin-containing membrane that could be used to assemble
disc membranes following ROS shedding. Whether there is rapid disc
membrane assembly in rat rods as there is in Xenopus is yet to be
established. There is no membrane assembly information available for
frogs, Rana pipiens, although it is known that opsin synthesis is
only slightly elevated when frogs are illuminated (Matsumoto and
Bok, 1979). However, Mercurio and Holtzman (1982a) have shown the
presence of subelliposoid smooth membranes in frog rods which are
also present throughout the elliposoid region and possibly represent
the same kind of membrane pool found in Xenopus and rats.

In vitro stimulation of phosphatidyl inositol synthesis by
light in rat retinas has been reported by Schmidt (1983) who also
found that the greatest amount of synthesis occurred in the micro-
dissected photoreceptor layer. This finding has been confirmed
autoradiographically in the present study and is in agreement with
the autoradiographic studies of Bibb and Young (1974) and Mercurio
and Holtzman (1982b) in frog. Based on sparse labeling of the outer
segments compared with intense labeling of the inner segments it
seems likely that much of the phospholipid isolated in the crude ROS
fraction in fact represents inner segment membranes which float with
ROS on sucrose solutions because of their similar polyunsaturated
fatty acid composition. These membranes might represent the precursor membranes discussed above.

These results differ from those of Anderson and Hollyfield
(1981) who observed light-stimulated synthesis of PI only in horizontal cells of Xenopus retinas using labeled inositol as a precursor. However, the use of labeled glycerol results in the labeling
of all the phospholipids in all cells and could easily mask a specific effect on PI in one cell type. Consequently, the failure to

observe such an effect cannot be taken as conclusive evidence.   A direct experiment with labeled inositol in rat retinas is required to resolve this apparent difference.

Further studies are planned to elucidate the biochemical events that occur during the requisite 2 hours of darkness and after the onset of light in light-triggered photoreceptor shedding in rats (Goldman, et al., 1980).

REFERENCES

Anderson, R.E., L.S. Feldman and G.L. Feldman. 1970.   Lipids of ocular tissues. II.   The phospholipids of mature bovine and rabbit whole retina.   Biochim. Biophys. Act 202: 367-373.

Anderson, R.E. and J.G. Hollyfield. 1981.   Light stimulates the incorporation of inositol into phosphatidylinositol in the retina.   Biochim. Biophys. Acta 665: 619-622.

Basinger, S., R. Hoffman and M. Matthes. 1976.   Photoreceptor shedding is initiated by light in the frog retina.   Science 194: 1074-1076.

Battelle, B.-A. and M.M. LaVail. 1980.   Protein synthesis in retinas of rats with inherited retinal dystrophy.   Exp. Eye Res. 31: 251-269.

Bergeron, J.J.M., R.A. Rachubinski, R.A. Sikstrom, B.I. Posner and J. Paiement. 1982.   Galactose transfer to endogenous acceptors within Golgi fractions of rat liver.   J. Cell Biol. 92: 139-146.

Besharse, J.C. 1982.   The daily light-dark cycle and rhythmic metabolism in the photoreceptor-pigment epithelium complex. In Progress in Retinal Research (N. Osborne and G. Chader, eds.). Pergammon Press, Oxford. pp81-124.

Besharse, J.C., J.G. Hollyfield and M.E. Rayborn, 1977a. Turnover of rod photoreceptor outer segments. II.   Membrane addition and loss in relationship to light.   J. Cell Biol. 75: 507-527.

Besharse, J.C., J.G. Hollyfield and M.E. Rayborn. 1977b. Photoreceptor outer segments: accelerated membrane renewal in rods after exposure to light.   Science 196: 536-538.

Bibb, C. and R.W. Young. 1974.   Renewal of glycerol in the visual cells and pigment epithelium of the frog retina.   J.Cell Biol. 62: 378-389.

Bligh, E.G. and W.J. Dyer. 1959.   A rapid method of total lipid extraction and purification.   Can. J. Biochem. Physiol. 37: 911-917.

Dudley, P.A. and P.J. O'Brien. 1981.   Circadian synthesis of rat retina membrane phospholipids.   Invest. Ophthalmol. Vis. Sci. 20 (Suppl.) 4.

Fairbanks, G., T.L. Steck and D.F.H. Wallach. 1971. Electrophoretic analysis of the major polypeptides of the human erythrocyte membrane.   Biochemistry. 10: 2606-2617.

Folch, J., M. Lees and G.H.S. Stanley. 1957.   A simple method for the isolation and purification of total lipids from animal tissues.   J. Biol. Chem. 226: 497-509.

Goldman, A.I., P.S. Teirstein and P.J. O'Brien. 1980.   The role of ambient lighting in circadian disc shedding in the rod outer segment of the rat retina.   Invest. Ophthalmol. Vis. Sci. 19: 1257-1267.

Gould, R.M. and R.M.C. Dawson. 1976.   Incorporation of newly formed lecithin into pheripheral nerve myelin.   J. Cell Biol. 68: 480-496.

Hollyfield, J.G. and S.F. Basinger. 1978. Photoreceptor shedding can be initiated within the eye. Nature 274: 794-796.

Hollyfield, J.G., J.C. Besharse and M.E. Rayborn. 1976. The effect of light on the quantity of phagosomes in the pigment epithelium. Exp. Eye Res. 23: 623-635.

Hollyfield, J.G., M.E. Rayborn, G.E. Verner, M.B. Maude and R.E. Anderson. 1982. Membrane addition to rod photoreceptor outer segments: light stimulates membrane assembly in the absence of increased membrane biosynthesis. Invest. Ophthalmol. Vis. Sci. 22: 417-427.

LaVail, M.M. 1976. Rod outer segment disc shedding in rat retina: relationship to cyclic lighting. Science 194: 1071-1073.

LaVail, M.M. 1980. Circadian nature of rod outer segment disc shedding in the rat. Invest. Ophthalmol. Vis. Sci. 19: 407-411.

Liang, C.J., K. Yamashita, C.G. Muellenberg, H. Shichi and A. Kobata. 1979. Structure of the carbohydrate moieties of bovine rhodopsin. J. Biol. Chem. 254: 6414-6418.

Lowry, O., N. Rosebrough, A. Farr and R. Randall. 1951. Protein measurement with the Folin phenol reagent. J. Biol. Chem. 193: 265-275.

Matusmoto, B. and D. Bok. 1979. Rhodopsin biosynthesis in Rana pipiens during the light-dark cycle. Invest. Ophthalmol. Vis. Sci. 18 (Suppl.) 267.

Mercurio, A.M. and E. Holtzman. 1982a. Smooth endoplasmic reticulum and other agranular reticulum in frog retinal photoreceptors. J. Neurocytol. 11: 263-293.

Mercurio, A.M. and E. Holtzman. 1982b. Ultrastructural localization of glycerolipid synthesis in rod cells of the isolated frog retina. J. Neurocytol. 11: 295-322.

O'Brien, P.J. and C.G. Muellenberg. 1968. Properties of glycosyl transfer enzymes of bovine retina. Biochim. Biophys. Acta 167: 268-273.

Papermaster, D.S. and B.G. Schneider. 1982. Biosynthesis and morphogenesis of outer segment membranes in vertebrate photoreceptor cells. In "Cell Biology of the Eye" D.S. McDevitt, ed. Academic Press, N.Y. pp. 475-531.

Papermaster, D.S., B.G. Schneider and J.C. Besharse. 1979. Assembly of rod photoreceptor membranes: Immunocytochemical and autoradiographic localization of opsin in smooth vesicles in the inner segment. J. Cell Biol. 83: 275a.

Rouser, G., A.N. Siakotos and S. Fleischer. 1966. Quantitative analysis of phospholipids by thin-layer chromatograph and phosphorus analysis of spots. Lipids 1: 85-86.

Schmidt, S.Y. 1983. Phosphatidylinositol synthesis and phosphorylation are enhanced by light in rat retinas. J. Biol. Chem. 258:6863-6868.

Teirstein, P.S., A.I. Goldman and P.J. O'Brien. 1980. Evidence for both local and central regulation of rat rod outer segment disc shedding. Invest. Ophthalmol. Vis. Sci. 19: 1268-1273.

Young, R.W. and D. Bok. 1969. Participation of the retinal pigment epithelium in the rod outer segment renewal process. J. Cell Biol. 42: 392-403.

Circadian Rhythms in Retinal Function

R.B. Barlow, S.C. Chamberlain, and L. Kass

The retina encodes and transmits information to the brain about the photic environment. In a number of animals the brain feeds back to the retina signals that modify the configuration of ganglion-cell receptive fields (Miles, 1970; Pearlman & Hughes, 1976), adapt the retina to changes in ambient illumination (Arechiga & Wiersma, 1969; Barlow et al, 1977; Fleissner & Fleissner, 1978; Levinson & Burnside, 1981; Yamashita & Tateda, 1981), or control metabolic processes in the retina (Chamberlain & Barlow, 1979; Teirstein et al, 1980). The efferent control of retinal function may be mediated by neural pathways or by circulating neurohormones.

The Limulus visual system provides a clear example of the efferent neural control of retinal function. Efferent fibers in the optic nerve trunk link the retina to a circadian clock located in the brain. The clock generates efferent activity at dusk, maintains the activity during the night, and stops the activity near dawn. No activity is recorded during the day. The daily rhythms in efferent activity continue unabated when the animal is maintained in constant darkness.

In this chapter we describe some of the effects the circadian clock exerts in the retina. In brief, we show that the efferent input mediates circadian rhythms in retinal response (Barlow et al., 1977; Barlow, 1983), increases the response and decreases the noise of the optic nerve discharge (Barlow et al., 1977), directly influences photoreceptor physiology (Kaplan & Barlow, 1980) and metabolism (Chamberlain & Barlow, 1979), changes the structure of retinal cells (Chamberlain & Barlow, 1977; Barlow & Chamberlain, 1980), increases the field of view of single ommatidia (Barlow et al, 1980), and decreases retinal inhibitory interactions (Batra & Barlow, 1982). We also discuss evidence that octopamine is a retinal neurotransmitter of the efferent effects (Kass & Barlow,

1980; Battelle et al., 1982;   Kass & Barlow, 1982).

EFFERENT OPTIC NERVE ACTIVITY MEDIATES CIRCADIAN RHYTHMS IN VISUAL
SENSITIVITY

When Limulus is kept in constant darkness, the lateral and
median eyes produce larger electroretinographic responses (ERGs) at
night than during the day. The seven-day experiment in figure 1
shows that the circadian rhythms are synchronous and that cutting
the optic nerve abolished the rhythms. At midnight of Day 3 the
recording cage was opened and a snare, which had been previously
placed around the left optic nerve trunk, was pulled to sever the
nerve. Cutting the nerve caused the amplitude of the ERG to fall
towards the low daytime level. The rate of fall approximates an
exponential function with a time constant of 0.78 hr. At midnight
on Days 5 and 7 the procedure was repeated for the median and right-
lateral optic nerves. In both cases the ERG amplitude decreased to
the daytime level and subsequent circadian changes in the ERG were
abolished.

The day-night changes in sensitivity which correspond to the
circadian changes in amplitude in figure 1 can be determined from
the function that relates ERG amplitude to the intensity of the
light flash. For all three records in figure 1 the changes in ERG
amplitude correspond to approximately a 20-fold change in sensitivity. Experiments with other animals yielded 20- to 100-fold
increases in sensitivity (Barlow, 1983).

Abolishing circadian rhythms by cutting the optic nerves in
figure 1 strongly suggests that the optic nerves transmit efferent
activity from a circadian clock located in the brain. Indeed, efferent activity can be recorded at night from the proximal stumps of
the cut optic nerves. Figure 2 shows trains of efferent activity
recorded simultaneously from the cut lateral optic nerves (median
nerve records are not shown). Note that only a single train of
efferent impulses could be recorded from the right optic nerve,
whereas regular bursts were recorded from the left optic nerve. The
efferent fibers are small, fragile, and often difficult to locate.
This and other experiments indicate that each lateral nerve contains
10 to 20 efferent fibers (Fahrenbach, 1971; Evans et al, 1982) which
fire in near synchrony with one another and with a group of efferent
fibers in the opposite lateral optic nerve.

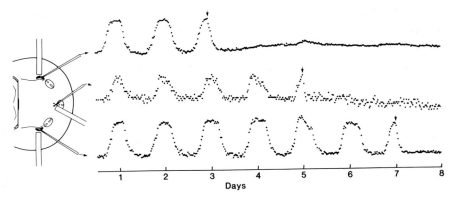

Figure 1. Circadian rhythms in the electroretinographic responses (ERGs) of the lateral eyes and median ocelli of Limulus. On the left is a diagram of the experimental preparation showing the location of the ERG electrodes. Also shown are the fiber-optic light pipes for delivering test flashes and the holes in the carapace for exposing the optic nerve trunks. Before the animal was placed in darkness, surgical snares were placed around each of the optic nerve trunks. On the right are plots of the peak-to-peak amplitude of the ERG in response to brief flashes delivered every 30 min for eight days while the animal remained in the dark. Arrows indicate the times at which the surgical snares were pulled to section the optic nerves. Note that each of the optic nerves is shown as sectioned in the diagram on the left. Before sectioning the optic nerves, the ERG of the lateral eyes exhibited circadian changes in amplitude from 40 µV during the day to 200 µV at night. Similarly the ERG of the median ocellus increased from 35 µV during the day to 120 µV at night. Taken from Barlow, 1983. Copyright 1983 by Williams and Wilkins Co.

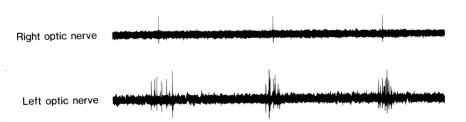

Figure 2. Efferent activity recorded at night from the right and left lateral optic nerves. Bursts of about nine spikes were recorded from the proximal stump of the cut left optic nerve, but only a single train of impulses was detected in the right optic nerve. The remaining efferent fibers in the right nerve may have been injured by dissection. It is apparent that efferent fibers in one nerve fire in synchrony with one another and with fibers in the opposite nerve. Recordings are 3.5 sec in duration. Taken from Barlow, 1983. Copyright 1983 by Williams and Wilkins Co.

Efferent optic nerve activity exhibits a circadian rhythm that is in phase with the circadian rhythm of the ERG amplitude (Barlow, 1982). Such a strong correlation between the endogenous efferent activity and the changes in ERG amplitude provides further evidence that efferent activity mediates the circadian changes in visual sensitivity. This possibility can be directly tested by "playing back" to the eye during the day the efferent activity recorded at night. This was done by triggering a current pulse generator with a train of efferent impulses previously recorded at night from the proximal stump of the cut optic nerve. Current pulses were delivered via a suction electrode to the distal stump of the cut optic nerve during the day. After four minutes of optic nerve stimultion, the ERG amplitude began to increase, and after one hour it reached the nighttime level (Barlow et al., 1977). In sum, pulses of current delivered to the cut optic nerve can mimic the effect of endogenous efferent activity on the ERG ampliude. We therefore conclude that efferent fibers in the optic nerve trunk mediate the circadian rhythms in visual sensitivity.

CIRCADIAN RHYTHM IN OPTIC NERVE DISCHARGE

Spontaneous and driven discharges of single optic nerve fibers also exhibit circadian rhythms (Barlow et al., 1977). The spike discharge of a single optic nerve fiber was recorded in situ with a glass suction electrode without cutting the optic nerve trunk or otherwise impairing the transmission of efferent activity from the brain to the eye. Once the appropriate recording was achieved, the eye was searched with a fiber-optic light pipe to locate and optically isolate the recorded ommatidium (Barlow, 1969). The preparation was then placed in a light-proof, shielded cage. Figure 3 (top) gives the steady-state rate of discharge to a brief flash of light delivered every hour for 56 hours while the animal remained in the dark. The results correspond to those for the ERG: high amplitude response at night and low during the day. Figure 3 (bottom) gives average rate of spontaneous activity recorded from the same optic nerve fiber during the periods between the hourly light flashes. The circadian rhythm in the light-evoked discharge of the optic nerve was expected, the circadian rhythm in spontaneous activity was not. One is the mirror image of the other. During the later evening hours the optic nerve responses were maximal and the spontaneous activity was minimal.

The circadian clock modulates retinal sensitivity in part by

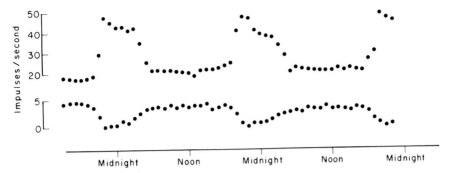

Figure 3. Circadian rhythms in the driven and spontaneous discharges of a single optic nerve fiber. Each of the upper points gives the mean firing rate of the dark-adapted ommatidium during the last 3 sec of a 6-sec flash presented every hour while the animal remained in the dark. The flash was presented via a light pipe which optically isolated the ommatidia and delivered 10^5 quanta per sec to the ommatidium at the cornea from 400 to 650 nm (corresponds to log I = -7 in figure 4). Each of the lower points gives the spontaneous activity of the ommatidium in a 25-sec interval in the dark. All points were recorded from the same optic nerve fiber. Taken from Barlow et al., 1977. Copyright 1977 by the American Association for the Advancement of Science.

changing the signal-to-noise ratio of the optic nerve discharge. If we define the driven discharge as the signal and the spontaneous activity as the noise which obscures the signal, then during the day the amplitude of the signal for the light intensity used in this experiment was approximately four times the amplitude of the noise. After midnight the signal-to-noise ratio increased more than tenfold. Before midnight the signal-to-noise ratio is difficult to define because near 10 P.M. no noise could be detected. We do not mean to imply that the clock's input abolishes all intrinsic retinal noise, but that it reduces the "dark" noise generated by the retina and transmitted to the brain.

The cellular mechanisms underlying the clock's influence on the light-evoked retinal responses are partially understood as discussed later in this chapter. The clock's influence on retinal noise can be traced to the photoreceptors as indicated in the following section.

The efferent input to the eye also influences the intensity coding characteristics of single ommatidia. Figure 4 gives the daytime and nighttime intensity-response function for the steady-state discharge recorded from a single optic nerve fiber in situ with the optic nerve uncut. This experiment followed the same procedure as that given in figure 3 except that here the optic nerve

36

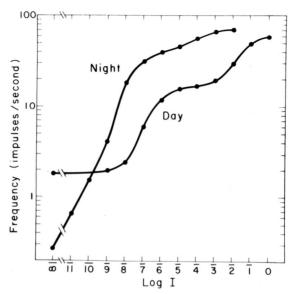

Figure 4. Intensity coding of a single ommatidium during the day and at night. The mean firing rate of a single optic nerve fiber during the last 3 sec of a 6-sec flash is plotted on the ordinate as a function of the logarithm of the relative light intensity plotted on the abscissa. The "day" intensity-response function was recorded from 3 to 4 P.M. and the "night" function from 9 to 10 P.M. The animal remained in the dark throughout the experiment. At log I = 0 approximately 10^{12} quanta per sec are incident on the ommatidium at the cornea from 400 to 650 nm. Taken from Barlow et al., 1977. Copyright 1977 by the American Association for the Advancement of Science.

response was recorded for a wide range of light intensities during the day and at night. The animal remained in the dark throughout the recording period, and the optically isolated ommatidium was allowed to dark adapt after each test flash.

Figure 4 shows that during the day the ommatidium exhibited a high spontaneous rate (~2 impulses/sec), a threshold for steady-state responses of about log I = -9, a graded response over at least a 9 log-unit range of light intensity, and a distinct plateau in response at intermediate intensities. These characteristics closely match those recorded from ommatidia in situ with the optic nerve cut (Barlow & Kaplan, 1971; Kaplan & Barlow, 1975). At night the same ommatidium exhibited a low spontaneous rate (0.2 impulses/sec), a threshold of less than log I = -11, a graded response over at least a 9 log-unit range, and no clear plateau at intermediate intensities.

Circadian changes in the position and the shape of the intensi-ty-response functions in figure 4 suggest changes in both the gain and the quantum catch of the retinal receptors. Subtracting the mean spontaneous rate from both functions shows that the daytime curve almost completely overlaps the nighttime curve if it is shifted 1.3 log units to the left and 0.5 log units vertically. A mismatch in the curves at high firing rates may result from saturation of the spike firing mechanism. Nevertheless, it appears that the action of the clock increases the photon catch by a factor of 20 and increases the gain by a factor of 3. As discussed below, circadian changes in ommatidial structure can readily account for changes in photon catch but not for changes in gain or spontaneous activity.

At night the threshold for eliciting steady-state optic nerve responses decreases about 2 log units. However, circadian changes in the shape of the intensity functions yield much greater changes in sensitivity for suprathreshold stimuli. For example, in figure 4 a steady-state optic nerve discharge of 20 impulses/sec requires 5 log units less light intensity at night than during the day.

CIRCADIAN RHYTHM IN PHOTORECEPTOR PHYSIOLOGY

The efferent input to the retina acts at an early stage in the process of visual excitation (Kaplan & Barlow, 1980). Figure 5 shows records of the membrane potential of a single dark-adapted photo-receptor (retinular cell) in situ. Each trace shows the membrane potential recorded in darkness for 20 sec and in response to a 5-sec flash of constant intensity. Recordings were made from 6 to 10 P.M. because previous experiments indicate that the efferent input from the clock to the retina begins in the early evening (~7 P.M.) and reaches maximal levels in the late evening (~10 P.M.).

At 6 P.M. discrete waves of membrane potential (quantum bumps) occurred in the dark and the response to the test flash was small. Later in the evening the discrete waves in the dark decreased in frequency and those in the light increased. At 9 and 10 P.M. no discrete waves occurred in the dark and the response to the test flash increased significantly. It appears that the clock's input to the retina decreases photoreceptor "noise" and increases photorecep-tor response.

The temporal changes in photoreceptor potential in figure 5 parallel those recorded from a single optic nerve fiber in figure 3. The photoreceptor potential is a fundamental component in the pro-cess of visual excitation. It represents the summation of discrete waves (Dodge et al., 1968) that are generated by the absorption of single photons (Yeandle, 1958; Adolph, 1964). Discrete waves

38

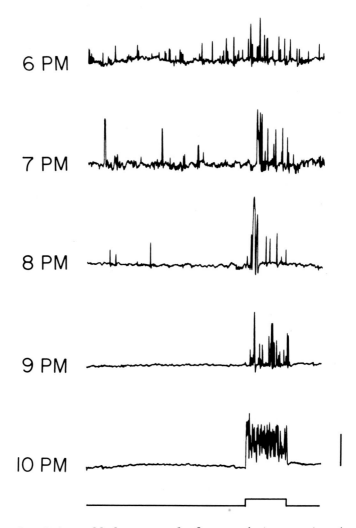

Figure 5. Intracellular records from a photoreceptor (retinular cell) in situ. The cell was impaled with a glass microelectrode at 4:30 P.M. and a light pipe was aligned on the cornea to optically isolate the ommatidium. The recording cage was closed at 5 P.M. to dark adapt the animal. Every hour during the next 5 hours, 5-sec flashes (bottom trace) were delivered to test the response of the cell. Each recording shows the membrane potential in darkness for 20 sec preceding the response to the test flash. Results of other experiments indicate that the circadian clock began to generate efferent optic nerve activity betwen 6 and 7 P.M. The efferent input abolished the occurrence of discrete waves in the dark by 9 P.M. and significantly increased the response to the test flash by 10 P.M. Cell resting potential was -50 mV. Scale bar, 10 mV. Taken from Kaplan and Barlow, 1980. Copyright 1980 by MacMillan Journals Limited.

occurring in the dark are thought to be caused by thermal events in the excitatory process (Adolph, 1968). These fluctuations in membrane potential are passively conducted from the retinal cells to the eccentric cell where they form the generator potential for spike initiation. Intracellular recordings in the dark reveal a direct correspondence between the discrete waves of retinular cells and the spontaneously occurring nerve impulses of eccentric cells (Barlow & Kaplan, 1977). Thus, it would appear reasonable to conclude that the decrease of the dark discharge of single optic nerve fibers (figure 3) orginates in the clock's reduction of discrete waves in the photoreceptor cells (figure 5). Likewise the nighttime increase in optic nerve discharge is caused by the nighttime increase in receptor potential.

The cellular mechanisms underlying the circadian changes in visual responses are not thoroughly understood. As indicated above, the nighttime increase in response can be attributed in part to an increase in the number of photons caught by the retinular cells. However, the nighttime reduction in photoreceptor noise cannot be attributed to any known cellular mechanism. If the spontaneously occurring discrete waves are, in fact, initiated by thermal events, by what mechanism does the efferent input to the retina abolish the effects of thermal energy without influencing those initiated by light?

No consistent changes in either the potential or resistance of the photoreceptor membrane were detected at the onset of efferent optic nerve activity. Moreover, light stimuli increased the frequency of discrete waves, not their ampltude (Figure 5). Thus the intracellular records from the photoreceptor cells do not reveal the origin of the increase in gain of the optic nerve discharge (Figure 4). Nevertheless the reduction of photoreceptor noise indicates that the efferent input to the retina acts at an early stage in the process of visual transduction.

CIRCADIAN RHYTHM IN THE STRUCTURE OF RETINAL CELLS

The circadian efferent input to the retina changes the morphology of the retinal cells (Chamberlain & Barlow, 1977; Barlow et al., 1980). Figure 6 shows reconstructions of dark-adapted ommatidia fixed during the day and at night. In the Limulus eye an ommatidium is composed of 8 to 12 retinular cells clustered tightly around the dendrite of an eccentric cell. Light collected by the corneal lens passes through an aperture formed by surrounding pig-

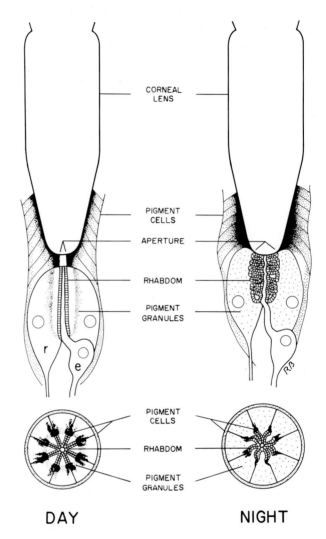

| CORNEAL LENS |
| PIGMENT CELLS |
| APERTURE |
| RHABDOM |
| PIGMENT GRANULES |
| PIGMENT CELLS |
| RHABDOM |
| PIGMENT GRANULES |

DAY   NIGHT

Figure 6.   Circadian changes in the morphology of a Limulus ommatidium.   Dark-adapted ommatidia were fixed in place during the day and
at night.   At the top are longitudinal reconstructions with the
plane of the section through the central ring of the rhabdom.
During the day the microvillus structure extends the entire length
of the eccentric-cell dendrite, whereas at night the rhabdom moves
distally toward the corneal lens causing deep folds in the
microvillus structure.   Shown at the bottom are cross-sectional
views taken halfway between the corneal lens and the eccentric-cell
body.   Each view shows eight retinular cells with their rhabdomeres
surrounding the eccentric-cell dendrite.   The width of the
microvillar structure was increased for diagrammatic purposes.   The
diameter of the corneal lens is 200 μm.   Taken from Barlow,
Chamberlain and Levinson, 1980. Copyright 1980 by the American
Association for the Advancement of Science.

ment cells and enters the photosensitive rhabdom of the retinular cells.

During the day the longitudinal reconstructions at the top of figure 6 show that the aperture formed by the distal pigment cells is constricted to about 17-μm diameter and the retinular cells are displaced from the tip of the lens by about 30 μm. These structural changes restrict the light entering the retinular cells. The cross-sectional view at the bottom shows processes of proximal pigment cells with large granules running between adjacent retinular cells at the ends of the rhabdomeral rays. Also, smaller pigment granules are concentrated in the cytoplasm of the retinular cells forming a circular band near the edge of the rhabdom.

At night the efferent input moves the processes of distal pigment cells away from the ommatidial axis and thereby increases the aperture diameter to 60 μm. The efferent input also shifts the retinular cells distally within 2 to 3 μm of the corneal lens. The cells appear to be compressed against the base of the lens inducing deep folds in the rhabdom and bends in the distal portion of the eccentric-cell dendrite. Processes of the proximal pigment cells recede and pigment granules within the retinular cells disperse. All morphological changes in figure 6 were obtained under conditions of complete dark adaptation. They continue in complete darkness, following the circadian rhythm of efferent optic nerve activity.

CIRCADIAN RHYTHM IN THE ACUITY OF LATERAL EYES

The circadian changes in morphology in figure 6 parallel changes in the field of view of single ommatidia (Barlow et al., 1980). The clock's effect on the field of view was determined with a fiber-optics light-pipe array attached to the arm of a vernier protractor at a distance of 20 cm from the cornea. Measurements of the threshold of the optic nerve discharge to brief flashes were made with the light pipe located at various angular positions along the anteroposterior axis of the eye. The acceptance angle (width of field of view at half maximum) was 6° during the day and 13° at night. Cutting the optic nerve abolishes the circadian changes in acceptance angle, leaving it in the narrow daytime state. Shocking the optic nerve during the day to mimic efferent activity increases the field of view to the nighttime state.

Circadian rhythms in the field of view can be largely attributed to circadian rhythms in ommatidial morphology. Precise measurements of the aperture and three-dimensional computer reconstructions of the rhabdom were utilized with a computer ray tracing program that models the refractive properties of the corneal lens (Fletcher et al, 1954; Land, 1979). Acceptance angles were calculated for both the daytime and nighttime structural states of dark-adapted ommatidia. The computed angle for the nighttime state closely matches the experimental measurement of 13°, but that for the daytime state is about one half the measured value of 6°. The discrepancy may result from light scatter by inhomogeneties within the corneal lenses. In any case, we feel that the refractile model of the ommatidium (Land, 1979) is valid and that the circadian rhythm in the field of view of the lateral eye results from morphological changes within the retinal photoreceptors.

Narrow fields of view of ommatidia during the day lower sensitivity but improve the resolution of spatial stimuli. Figure 7 shows the acceptance angles for three ommatidia located in a horizontal line near the center of the eye. Ommatidia 1 and 2 are separated by 1.5 receptor diameters and their optic axes diverge by 10°. Ommatidia 2 and 3 are separated by two diameters, and their axes diverge by 12°. In this region of the retina the optic axes of adjacent ommatidia diverge by approximately 5°, which is about equal to the daytime acceptance angles of each of the ommatidia. Thus, during the day when ambient illumination is high, each ommatidium "sees" approximately its proportional share of visual space.

At night the wide fields of view increase sensitivity and reduce spatial resolution. The nighttime acceptance angles for ommatidia 1,2, and 3 are 10.8^O, 13.7^O, and 12° respectively. Since these angles are about twice those separating the optic axes of adjacent ommatidia, the fields of view of adjacent ommatidia overlap considerably. A distant point source of light on the optic axis of one ommatidium would appear about 80% less intense to a neighboring receptor during the day, but only about 50% less intense at night. Thus under control of a circadian clock the Limulus eye exchanges its daytime acuity for greater sensitivity at night.

CIRCADIAN RHYTHM IN LATERAL INHIBITION

The efferent input to the retina at night decreases the strength of the lateral inhibitory interactions exerted among neighboring ommatidia (Batra & Barlow, 1982). The effects of such circadian changes in inhibition were detected in the pattern of optic nerve response generated by a simple step pattern of illumination on the retina. It is well known that lateral inhibition enhances such patterns by producing maxima and minima in response near the border (Ratliff & Hartline, 1959; Barlow & Quarles, 1975). These maxima and minima are physiological correlates of Mach bands. The width of the Mach bands is related to the configuration of the inhibitory field (Barlow & Quarles, 1975). The efferent input to the retina at

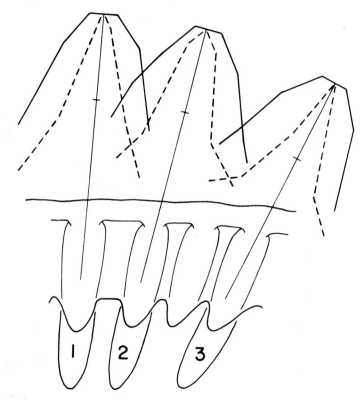

Figure 7. Acceptance angles for three ommatidia located along a horizontal line in the center of the eye. The curves at the top give the relative sensitivity of the optic nerve discharge for each recorded ommatidia plotted on a linear scale as a function of the angle of incidence of test flashes delivered from a point light source. For comparison the nighttime (solid line) and daytime (broken line) measurements are normalized to a value of 1.0 at the point of peak sensitivity. The widths of the acceptance angle at 0.5 sensitivity (cross ticks on optic axis) for ommatidia 1,2, and 3 are 10.8°, 13.7°, and 12° at night and 5.4°, 6.5°, and 5.1° during the day. The recorded ommatidia were about fifty times more sensitive at night than during the day for point light sources lying along the optic axes. The longitudinal reconstruction showing the relative position and orientation of the three recorded ommatidia is based on light micrographs of the lateral eye which was marked and prepared for sectioning after the physiological recording was terminated. Ommatidia 1 and 2 do not lie adjacent to one another but are separated by 1.5 receptor diameters. Their optic axes diverge by 10°. Likewise, ommatidia 2 and 3 are separated by 2 receptor diameters, and their optic axes diverge by 12°.

night shifts the Mach-band pattern to higher response levels without significantly changing the shape or width of the Mach bands. This result was obtained after the overall level of illumination of the retina was reduced to compensate for the nighttime increase in retinal sensitivity. Apparently the clock's input to the retina decreases the strength of lateral inhibitory interactions without changing the configuration of the inhibitory field. Perhaps the increased strength of inhibition during the day serves to maintain contrast enhancement under bright ambient illumination without saturation of optic nerve responses.

Modulation of the strength of lateral inhibition by the circadian clock has an anatomical basis. W. H. Fahrenbach (personal communication) has found abundant synaptic contacts of efferent terminals on collateral branches which mediate the inhibitory interactions in the retina.

Regarding the possible consequences of circadian rhythms in excitation and inhibition, it is interesting to note that, under appropriate conditions, the optic nerve fibers discharge impulses in synchronized bursts (Renninger & Barlow, 1979; 1980). This is especially true at night when sustained bursts of nerve impulses can be detected over a wide range of incident light intensities. The role of such bursting activity is not clear, but measurements of optical transmission in coastal seawater indicate that at depths of up to 10 meters the downwelling illumination from moonlight is sufficient to trigger the synchronized optic nerve responses.

SHORT-TERM AND LONG-TERM EFFECTS OF THE EFFERENT INPUT TO THE RETINA

The endogenous nighttime changes in retinal anatomy and physiology described thus far have one common characteristic: they can be reproduced during the day by applying current pulses to the optic nerve trunk. These striking changes begin within minutes of the onset of optic nerve shock and reach full amplitude within one hour. After cessation of nerve shock the retina returns to the daytime state following an exponential function with a time constant of 0.78 hr. Blocking the efferent input from the clock at night by sectioning the optic nerve causes the same rate of return to the daytime state (see figure 1).

The circadian clock exerts additional effects on the retina that cannot be reproduced by short periods of optic nerve shock. Several aspects of retinal function in Limulus require long-term efferent input from the clock. As described below, the daily turnover of rhodopsin containing membrane at the first light of dawn requires an extended period of efferent input the preceding night (Chamberlain & Barlow, 1979). Also described below is the requirement of efferent activity for photomechanical changes in the retina. In both cases an extended period of efferent activity is required before the light-initiated retinal process takes place. The efferent input appears to prime the retina for these processes rather than generate them.

EFFERENT CONTROL OF PHOTORECEPTOR MEMBRANE TURNOVER

Efferent optic nerve activity and light controls the daily turnover of rhabdom in the photoreceptor cells of the Limulus lateral eye (Chamberlain & Barlow, 1979). The photosensitive membrane structures are broken down and rebuilt at the first light onset each day. Figure 8 shows the sequence of light-induced changes in the

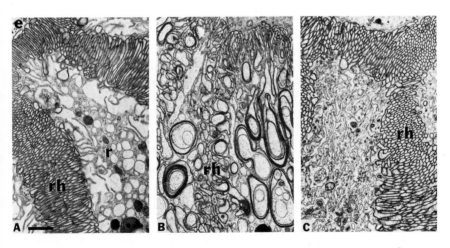

Figure 8. Rhabdom turnover in Limulus photoreceptors. Electron micrographs show the temporal sequence of breakdown and renewal of photosensitive membrane structures in retinular cells. (A) Part of the rhabdom of a lateral eye of an animal not exposed to light. The microvillar array of the rhabdomeres (rh) of adjacent retinular cells is also present at the border between the eccentric cell dendrite (e) and the retinular cell (r). (B) Breakdown of the rhabdom after 15 minutes of continous exposure to sunlight. The microvillar array is disrupted and much of its membrane has been incorporated into lamellar bodies. (C) Renewal of the rhabdom after 30 minutes of continous exposure to light. The microvillar array has been reconstructed and numerous multivesicular bodies have formed from the lamellar bodies. Bar represents 1 μm. Taken from Chamberlain and Barlow, 1979. Copyright 1979 by the American Association for the Advancement of Science.

rhabdomeres of the retinular cells. Figure 8A shows a partial cross section of the rhabdom from the eye of an animal that was maintained in darkness through the night and was fixed in darkness the following day. Well-defined microvillar arrays from positions of the rhabdomeres of three adjacent retinular cells are visible. The procedure for figure 8B was the same as for figure 8A except that the animal was exposed for 15 minutes before the fixative was injected into the eye. The rays of the rhabdom are almost completely disassembled by the brief exposure, and whorls of microvillar membrane have formed lamellar bodies. Figure 8C shows a third animal that was exposed to 30 minutes of sunlight before fixation. The rhabdom is nearly restored to its original state, thus the entire breakdown and reassembly process is complete within 30 minutes.

Blocking the efferent input to the retina blocks the turnover of photoreceptive membrane. Efferent activity must precede the light-initiated turnover, but the efferent optic nerve fibers need not be active when turnover occurs. The amount of efferent activity required to prime rhabdom turnover was roughly estimated by exposing the eye at various times during the night. No turnover was detected until the retina had received 3 to 5 hours of efferent input.

Mimicking the efferent input to the retina restores membrane turnover. In one experiment both lateral optic nerve trunks were sectioned, and the distal end of one cut nerve trunk was pulled into a suction electrode. As described above for the ERG experiments, efferent activity of the type shown in figure 2 was "played back" to the eye via the suction electrode. After 8 hours of optic nerve stimulation the animal was exposed to light, and the eyes were fixed 15 minutes later. The rhabdoms of the eye receiving artificial efferent input turned over, the rhabdoms of the fellow eye did not.

Membrane turnover was also investigated under conditions of natural diurnal illumination. Animals were freshly collected and fixed at various times over a 24-hour period in the month of June. Transient turnover occurred at the very first light of dawn between the hours of 4 to 5 A.M. The turnover occurred over a period of about 30 minutes and represented a fourfold decrease in membrane area. At that time of the day the efferent optic nerve fibers are still active and the retina is in the nighttime state, both physiologically and anatomically. In spite of these differences, the rhabdom turnover did not differ appreciably in time course or in ultrastructural appearance from that carried out later in the day under laboratory conditions. Although little is known of the cellu-

lar mechanism involved in priming and triggering turnover, it is
clear that both light and efferent input from circadian clock are
involved.

EFFERENT CONTROL OF PHOTOMECHANICAL CHANGES

Retinal cells exhibit circadian rhythms in morphology under
conditions of complete darkness (figure 7). Exposure to diurnal
lighting enhances the circadian changes in morphology. Under conditions of natural ambient illumination, the retinular cells continue
to move away from the tip of the corneal lens, reaching a distance
of about 80 μm by late afternoon. Also, the ratio of rhadom length
to width increases from 1.2 at night to 4.0 during the day under
diurnal lighting, whereas under constant darkness (figure 6), the
ratio only changes from 1.2 to 2.6. Thus, under conditions of
natural daylight the photosensitive structure of the receptor cells
becomes long, thin, and far removed from the corneal lens.

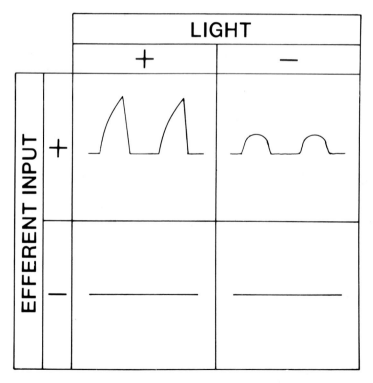

Figure 9. Summary of the interplay of circadian efferent activity
and diurnal lighting in producing rhythms in lateral eye structure.
Efferent input to the retina produces circadian changes in structure
which are enhanced by diurnal lighting. Diurnal lighting alone has
no effect.

Diurnal lighting alone has no effect on ommatidial morphology. If the endogenous efferent input to the retina is chronically blocked by cutting the optic nerve, no morphological changes will occur that are correlated with diurnal lighting. As described above for rhabdom turnover, the efferent input appears to prime the retina for subsequent photomechanical changes. Figure 9 summarizes the interaction of efferent activity and diurnal lighting.

Cellular mechanisms underlying the changes in retinal morphology have not been studied in detail. However, preliminary evidence indicates that microtubules and microfilaments may be involved. At night, injection behind the cornea of a microtubular inhibitor, vinblastine, decreases retinal sensitivity and changes retinal morphology toward the daytime state. During the day the same injection increases retinal sensitivity and changes retinal morphology toward the nighttime state. Both injections produce approximately the same sensitivity levels and morphological changes which are intermediate to the normal daytime and nighttime states. Cytochalasin B, the microfilament inhibitor, produced similar results. Apparently the daytime state of low sensitivity, as well as the nighttime state of high sensitivity, requires the integrity of cytoskeletal structures in the retinal cells.

Figure 10 summarizes the structural changes exerted by the circadian clock. Figure 10A shows the structural parts of the ommatidia and figure 10B indicates some of the changes that occur at night. The drawings are reconstructed from serial cross sections. The efferent fibers were added to indicate schematically that each type of cell within the ommatidium is contacted by efferent terminals (Fahrenbach, 1981).

OCTOPAMINE: AN EFFERENT NEUROTRANSMITTER

The efferent input to the retina exerts a multiplicity of physiological and anatomical effects without detectable changes in the membrane potential or membrane resistance of retinal cells. This is not characteristic of conventional chemical synaptic transmission, but may be indicative of a neurohormonal or neurosecretory process. In an attempt to identify the efferent neurotransmitter we injected beneath the cornea small aliquots of a wide variety of candidates. Octopamine met all five criteria for a neurotransmitter: synthesis, localization, release (Battelle et al., 1982; Evans et al., 1983), physiological mimicry, and pharmacological blockade

(Kass & Barlow, 1980, 1982). We should qualify this statement by noting that injection of octopamine (10 μM) during the day increased retinal sensitivity and changed retinal structure toward the nighttime state, but rarely achieved a complete conversion. It is possible that our method of injection does not adequately mimic the natural state or that octopamine does not act alone.

Injection at night of clozapine (25 μM), a demonstrated antagonist of octopamine, reversibly decreases retinal sensitivity. Also, both dibutryryl-cAMP (1 mM) and forskolin (40 μM) increase retinal sensitivity and change retinal structure to the nighttime state when injected during the day. Forskolin activates adenylate cyclase and dB-cAMP penetrates cell membranes and can substitute for cAMP's action on protein kinases. Both results suggest that efferent neurotransmission in the Limulus retina may be yet another example of cAMP serving as a second messenger in synaptic processes of the long-time base type (Greengard, 1975; Nathanson, 1977).

Figure 11 presents a proposed scheme for the neurochemistry of the efferent effects on the retinal photoreceptors. We have as yet no firm evidence regarding the efferent effects on other retinal

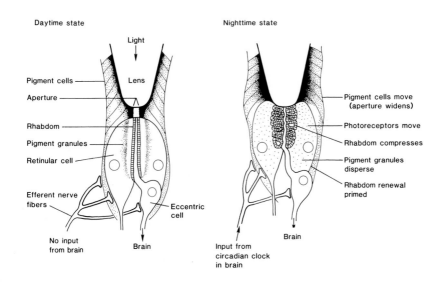

Figure 10. Summary of structural changes in the retina produced by the circadian clock. The reconstruction on the left shows the component of the ommatidium in the daytime state. The efferent nerve terminals are schematic. They were included to indicate that each cell type of the ommatidium receives synaptic input from the circadian clock (Fahrenbach, 1981). On the right are shown the various structural changes that are either initiated or primed by the clock's input.

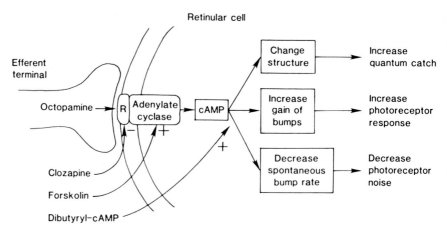

Figure 11. Proposed scheme for the neurochemistry of the circadian efferent input on photoreceptor cells.

cells. Also, we have no evidence regarding the role of octopamine in the long-term effects (rhabdom turnover and photomechanical changes) of the efferent input to the retina.

SUMMARY

The circadian clock in the Limulus brain is a fundamental component of the visual system. At night it transmits efferent optic nerve activity to the lateral eyes, median ocelli, and ventral photoreceptors (Eisele et al., 1982). As described in this chapter, the efferent input to the lateral eyes exerts multiple physiological and anatomical effects that combine to increase retinal sensitivity. The efferent input to the median ocelli increases their sensitivity in the visible range, but not in the ultraviolet, to which they are most sensitive (Barlow et al, 1980). The efferent input to the ventral photoreceptors has no known effect (Kaplan et al, 1980). The clock's influence on the lateral eye can be divided into short-term and long-term effects. The short-term effects, initiated by the onset of efferent activity at night, increase retinal sensitivity. The long-term effects, primed by preceding efferent activity, control retinal metabolism and enable the retina to adapt to high levels of illumination during the day. Although our knowledge of the visual system is far from complete (Chamberlain & Barlow, 1980, 1982), it is clear that the animals have evolved numerous mechanisms for adapting visual sensitivity to fluctuations in ambient illumination caused by the earth's rotation.

Behavioral studies show that the animal's sensitivity to light fluctuates from day to night (Powers & Barlow, 1981). A classical conditioning procedure using movements of the tail and gill yielded a change in behavioral threshold that corresponds in magnitude to the changes in physiological threshold reported in this chapter. In addition, a study of Limulus mating behavior was carried out using cement castings of the female carapace and other forms (Barlow et al., 1982). In the spring, crabs congregate to build nests on protected beaches near the water's edge at high tide. The mating activity is most pronounced at night. Observations show that males are attracted to the painted cement castings, the degree of attraction depending on the form and contrast of the castings, and on the time of day. Since the discrimination of contrast requires vision, it is possible that the high visual sensitivity generated at night by the circadian clock may adapt the animal for nocturnal mating behavior.

ACKNOWLEDGEMENTS

This research was supported by NSF grant BNS-8104669 and NIH grants EY-00667, EY-03446, and EY-05443.

REFERENCES

Adolph, A.R. 1964. Spontaneous slow potential fluctuations in the Limulus photoreceptor. J. Gen. Physiol. 48: 297-322.

Adolph, A.R. 1968. Thermal and spectral sensitivities of discrete slow potentials in Limulus eye. J. Gen. Physiol. 52: 584-599.

Arechiga, H. and C.A.G. Wiersma. 1969. Circadian rhythm of responsiveness in crayfish visual units. J. Neurobiol. 1: 71-85.

Barlow, R.B., Jr. 1969. Inhibitory fields in the Limulus lateral eye. J. Gen. Physiol. 54: 383-396.

Barlow, R.B., Jr. 1983. Carcadian rhythms in the Limulus visual system. J. Neurosci. 3:856-870.

Barlow, R.B., Jr., S.J. Bolanowski and M.L. Brachman. 1977. Efferent optic nerve fibers mediate circadian rhythms in the Limulus eye. Science 197: 86-89.

Barlow, R.B., Jr. and S.C. Chamberlain. 1980. Light and a circadian clock modulate structure and function in Limulus photoreceptors. In: The Effects of Constant Light on Visual Processes. T.P. Williams and B.N. Baker (Eds.), Plenum, New York, pp. 247-269.

Barlow, R.B., Jr., S.C. Chamberlain, S.J. Bolanowski, Jr., L.A. Galway, Jr. and D.P. Joseph. 1980. One eye can increase the sensitivity of another in Limulus. Soc. Neurosci. Abstr. 6: 344.

Barlow, R.B., Jr., S.C. Chamberlain, and J.Z. Levinson. 1980. Limulus brain modulates the structure and function of the lateral eyes. Science 210: 1037-1039.

Barlow, R.B., Jr. and E. Kaplan. 1971. Limulus lateral eye: properties of receptor units in the unexcised eye. Science 174: 1027-1029.

Barlow, R.B., Jr. and E. Kaplan. 1977. Properties of visual cells in the lateral eye of Limulus in situ. J. Gen. Physiol. 69: 203-220.

Barlow, R.B., Jr., L.C. Ireland and L. Kass. 1982. Vision has a role in Limulus mating behaviour. Nature 296: 65-66.

Barlow, R.B., Jr. and D.A. Quarles, Jr. 1975. Mach bands in the lateral eye of Limulus: comparison of theory and experiment. J. Gen. Physiol. 65: 709-730.

Batra, R. and R.B. Barlow, Jr. 1982. Efferent control of pattern vision in Limulus. Soc. Neurosci. Abstr. 8: 49.

Battelle, B.-A., J.A. Evans and S.C. Chamberlain. 1982. Efferent fibers to Limulus eyes synthesize and release octopamine. Science 216: 1250-1252.

Chamberlain, S.C. and R.B. Barlow, Jr. 1977. Morphologial correlates of efferent circadian activity and light adaptation in the Limulus lateral eye. Biol. Bull. 153: 418-419.

Chamberlain, S.C. and R.B. Barlow, Jr. 1979. Light and efferent activity control rhabdom turnover in Limulus photoreceptors. Science 206: 361-363.

Chamberlain, S.C. and R.B. Barlow, Jr. 1980. Neuroanatomy of the visual afferents in the horseshoe crab (Limulus polyphemus). J. Comp. Neurol. 192: 387-400.

Chamberlain, S.C. and R.B. Barlow, Jr. 1982. Retinotopic organization of lateral eye input to Limulus brain. J. Neurophysiol. 48: 505-520.

Dodge, F.A., Jr., B.W. Knight and J. Toyoda. 1968. Voltage noise in Limulus visual cells. Science 160: 88-90.

Eisele, L.E., L. Kass and R.B. Barlow, Jr. 1982. Circadian clock generates optic nerve activity in the excised Limulus brain. Biol. Bull. 163: 382.

Evans, J.A., B.-A. Battelle and S.C. Chamberlain. 1983. Audioradiographic localization of newly synthesized octopamine to retinal efferents in the Limulus visual system. J. Comp. Neurol. (in press).

Fahrenbach, W.H. 1971. The morphology of the Limulus visual system. IV. The lateral optic nerve. Z. Zellforsch. 114: 532-545.

Fahrenbach, W.H. 1981. The morphology of the Limulus visual system. VII. Innervation of photoreceptor neurons by neurosecretory efferents. Cell Tissue Res. 216: 655-659.

Fleissner, G., and G. Fleissner. 1978. The optic nerve mediates the circadian pigment migration in the median eyes of the scorpion. Comp. Biochem. Physiol. 61: 69-71.

Fletchner, A., T. Murphy and A. Young. 1954. Solutions of two optical problems. Proc. Roy. Soc. Lond. 223: 216-225.

Greengard, P. 1975. Cyclic nucleotides, protein phosphorylation and neuronal function. Advanc. Cyclic Nucleotide Res. 5: 585-602.

Kaplan, E. and R.B. Barlow, Jr. 1975. Properties of visual cells in the lateral eye of Limulus in situ: extracellular recordings. J. Gen. Physiol. 66: 303-326.

Kaplan, E. and R.B. Barlow, Jr. 1980. Circadian clock in Limulus brain increases response and decreases noise of retinal photoreceptors. Nature 286: 393-395.

Kaplan, E., R. Batra and R.B. Barlow, Jr. 1980. Recording from the Limulus ventral eye in situ: Is there a circadian rhythm? Biol. Bull. 159: 486.

Kass, L. and R.B. Barlow, Jr. 1980. Octopamine increases the ERG of the Limulus lateral eye. Biol. Bull. 159: 487.

Kass, L. and R.B. Barlow, Jr. 1982. Efferent neurotransmission of circadian rhythms in Limulus lateral eye: single cell studies. Biol. Bull. 163: 386.

Land, M.F. 1979. The optical mechanism of the eye of Limulus. Nature 280:396-397.

Levinson, G. and Burnside, B. 1981. Circadian rhythms in teleost retinomotor movements. A comparison of the effects of circadian rhythm and light condition on cone length. Invest. Ophthalmol. Vis. Sci. 20: 294-303.

Miles, F.A. 1970. Centrifugal effects in the avian retina. Science 170: 992-995.

Nathanson, J.A. 1977. Cyclic nucleotides and nervous system function. Physisol. Rev. 57: 157-256.

Pearlman, A.L. and C.P. Hughes. 1976. Functional role of efferents to the avian retina. II. Effects of reversible cooling of the isothmo-optic nucleus. J. Comp. Physiol. 166: 123-132.

Powers, M.K. and R.B. Barlow, Jr. 1981. Circadian changes in visual sensitivity of Limulus: behavioral evidence. Biol. Bull. 161: 350.

Ratliff, F. and H.K. Hartline. 1959. The responses of Limulus optic nerve fibers to patterns of illumination of the receptor mosaic. J. Gen. Physiol. 42: 1241-1255.

Renninger, G.H. and R.B. Barlow, Jr. 1979. Lateral inhibition, excitation, and the circadian rhythm of the Limulus compound eye. Soc. Neurosci. Abstr. 5: 804.

Renninger, G.H. and R.B. Barlow, Jr. 1980. Lateral inhibition can synchronize optic-nerve impulses. Topical Meeting on Recent Advances in Vision. Opt. Soc. Am., Apr. 30 to May 3, 1980.

Teirstein, P.S., A.I. Goldman and P.J. O'Brien. 1980. Evidence for both local and central regulation of rat rod out segment disc shedding. Invest. Ophthalmol. Vis. Sci. 19: 1268-1273.

Yamashita, S. and H. Tateda. 1981. Efferent neural control in the eyes of orb weaving spiders. J. Comp. Physiol. 143: 477-483.

Yeandle, S. 1958. Evidence of quantized slow potentials in the eye of Limulus. Am. J. Ophthalmol. 463, Part II (Sept.).

Cone Pathways in the Mammalian Retina

H. Kolb

The basic neurocircuitry underlying the highest visual acuity pathways in such animals as birds, primates and certain reptiles (Cajal, 1933) is thought to consist of a bipolar cell/ganglion cell chain connected in a one to one fashion with a single cone photoreceptor. In the monkey retina, for example, there are midget bipolar cells and midget ganglion cells that subserve an individual cone (Polyak, 1941), In 1969 it was reported that the cone midget bipolar pathways of the rhesus monkey retina consisted of a pair of bipolars characterized by different types of synaptic contact with the cone pedicles in the outer plexiform layer (OPL) (Kolb et al., 1969). One of the midget bipolars inserted dendritic terminals into the synaptic complex of the cone pedicle to make "invaginating" contacts beneath the synaptic ribbon (Figures 1,2). The other midget bipolar, in contrast, made synaptic contacts with the surface of the cone pedicle on either side of the invaginating elements (Figures 1,3). In addition the two midget bipolar types were found to have different termination levels of their axons in the inner plexiform layer (IPL). The flat midget bipolar (fmb) had a club-shaped axon terminal that ended in neuropil closest to the row of amacrine cell bodies on the outer limit of the IPL, while the invaginating midget bipolar (imb) had an axon terminal penetrating to neuropil closer to the ganglion cells (Figure. 4 fmb axon ends in a, while imb axon ends in b). Kolb (1970) suggested that the two levels of ending of the two varieties of midget bipolar was correlated with the two different branching levels of the midget ganglion cells that Polyak (1941) had noted and remarked upon. Gouras (1971) further suggested that as ganglion cells of the monkey fovea had either ON center or OFF center receptive field physiology, the midget bipolar to midget ganglion cell chain was organized into one using invaginating midget bipolars to subserve ON center pathway and

the other, using flat midget bipolars, for OFF center pathways
Interestingly, Marr (1974) also modelled ON center and OFF center
channels for the primate retina with the midget bipolar/ganglion
cell chain but he reversed the roles of the bipolars as originating
ON and OFF center responses.

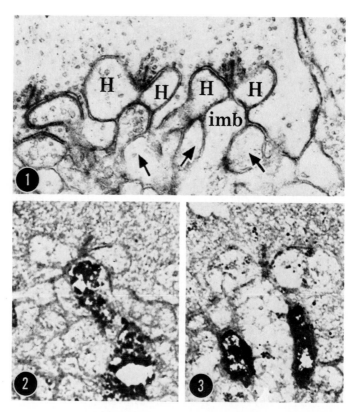

Figures 1-3:   Electron micrographs of synaptic junctions between a
cone pedicle and bipolar and horizontal cell dendrites in the rhesus
monkey retina. Figure 1: General morphology of the cone pedicle
synapses.   The invaginating synapses consist of a triad of processes
postsynaptic to cone pedicle ribbons.   Lateral elements (H) are from
horizontal cells and the central elements (imb) from invaginating
midget bipolars for the most part. Arrows indicate synaptic contacts of flat midget bipolar cells at semi-invaginating basal junctions, X 22,800. Figure 2: Golgi-impregnated dendrite of an invaginating midget bipolar cell forming the central element of the
triad at the ribbon synapse, X 23,000. Figure 3: Golgi-impregnated
dendrites of a flat midget bipolar ending at semi-invaginating basal
junctions, X 30,000. Modified from Kolb et al., (1969).

It appears then, that the rhesus monkey has at least a double output from the single cone photoreceptor assuming that all cones make contact with both midget bipolar types. The hypothesis is that the double output is to ensure parallel ON center and OFF center channels for each cone to the brain. Proving this hypothesis in rhesus monkey retina, however, needs the confirmatory evidence of intracellular recordings of light responses from both midget ganglion cells. These kinds of experiments have not yet been possible in the monkey retina. Instead one must draw parallels from evidence attained on the neurocircuitry of another mammalian retina, the cat retina, where such functional anatomy is now becoming available.

The cat retina does not have a single channel midget bipolar cell system and neither does it have a rod-free central foveola where the highest concentration of specialized cones initiates the high acuity pathways, typical of the higher primates. However, the area centralis of the cat retina has the lowest ratio of cones to a ganglion cell (5:1) (Steinberg et al., 1973), and is, thus, considered to be the high acuity specialization of the cat retina. In actual fact, the structure and neural connections of the area centralis of the cat are probably equivalent to perifoveal regions of rhesus retina (Polyak, 1941). In the area centralis of cat retina can be found the bipolar cells and ganglion cells with the smallest dendritic trees (Boycott and Kolb, 1973; Boycott and Wässle, 1974; Kolb et al., 1981), which are thought to form the components of the high acuity system of the cat.

BIPOLAR CELLS

Comparison of Figures 4 and 5, where drawings of Golgi-impregnated bipolar cells of the rhesus monkey and the cat retina are shown, indicates the similarities between the bipolar cells of the two species. Both species have only a single type of rod bipolar (rb) which had similar types of synaptic contacts with rod spherules (invaginating, ribbon related) (Kolb, 1970; Boycott and Kolb, 1973), and similar appearing axon terminals that end deep in the IPL close to the ganglion cell layer (b in Figures 4 and 5). Cone bipolars, on the other hand, are of several different morphological varieties in both species. In addition to the two midget bipolar types, the rhesus monkey has a diffuse flat bipolar (dfb) (Polyak, 1941; Boycott and Dowling, 1969; Kolb, 1970) and a diffuse invaginating bipolar (dib) (Polyak, 1941; Mariani, 1981). Furthermore, there are reported to be single-cone-contacting, non-midget bipolars and

58

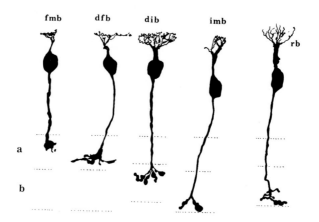

fmb   dfb   dib   imb   rb

a

b

Figure 4: Camera lucida drawings of bipolar cells in the rhesus
monkey retina from peri-foveal retina. The flat midget bipolar
(fmb) and the invaginating midget bipolar (imb) contact only a
single cone. They are distinguished by the level of ending of their
axon terminals in the IPL, a for fmb and b for imb. The diffuse
cone bipolar contacts approximately seven cones and the diffuse flat
bipolar (dfb) has an axon ending in a of the IPL while the diffuse
invaginating bipolar (dib) has an axon ending in b of the IPL. The
rod bipolar (rb) contacts 15-30 rods and has an axon ending deep in
b of the IPL.

giant bistratified bipolar cells in rhesus monkey retina (Mariani,
1982) (not illustrated on Figure. 4).

    The bipolar cells of the cat retina are all diffuse in that
they contact more than one cone (Figure 5). However, some varieties
of cone bipolar are narrower-field than others so they end up contacting fewer cones than other varieties. The three narrow-field
varieties are cbl, cb5 and cb6 (Boycott and Kolb, 1973; Kolb et al.,
1981). These cell types all have a similar-appearing, small
dendritic spread, contacting between 4 and 8 cones in the area
centralis. Their axon terminals distinguish them though. The cbl
bipolar has a compact varicose intertwined group of axon branches
that ramify in neuropil just below the amacrine cell bodies (sublamina a; Famiglietti and Kolb, 1976) (Figure 5), while cb5 has a
vertically penetrating axon terminal consisting of varicosities
stretching through the lower IPL (sublamina b; Famiglietti and Kolb,
1976). Cb6, on the other hand, has a laterally spreading axon lying
in S3 (Cajal, 1933) or the middle of sublamina b (Figure. 5). The
other cone bipolar cell types of the cat retina, of which only three
are shown in Figure 5 (Kolb et al., 1981), have wider dendritic
spreads and markedly stratified axon terminals in the IPL. Cb2 has

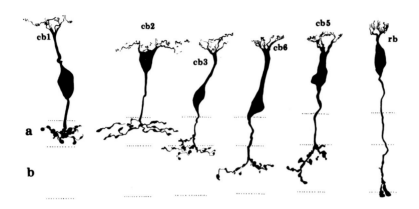

Figure 5: Camera lucida drawings of Golgi-impregnated bipolar cells of central cat retina (within 1mm of the area centralis). Cb1, cb5 and cb6 are narrow-field bipolar cells that contact 4-8 cones. Their axon termination distinguish them. Cb1 has an axon terminal ending in sublamina a of the IPL while cb5 and cb6 have axons of differing morphology ending in b of the IPL. Cb2 is a wider field bipolar that has a laterally spreading axon in a of the IPL and cb3 has its axon straddling the a/b border. The rod bipolar contacts approximately 15 cones and has an axon ending deep in b of the IPL.

a laterally coursing, beaded axon running in S2 of Cajal's (1933) scheme, or lower sublamina a of Famiglietti and Kolb's (1976) scheme. Cb3 has an axon terminal that straddles the sublamina a/sublamina b border.

Because of the narrow-field nature of cb1, cb5 and cb6 it seems intuitively likely that they are the equivalent of the flat and invaginating midget bipolar cells of monkey retina in some way. Clearly cb1 and the flat midget would be considered equivalent (Boycott and Kolb, 1973) but which of cb5 or cb6 is equivalent to the invaginating midget of rhesus retina? Some answer to this question may come with knowledge of the type of synapse these bipolars form with the cone pedicles, their intracellular photoresponses, and the nature of their connections with ganglion cells.

Intracellular recordings and staining with horseradish peroxidase (HRP) have been possible in several of the cone bipolar types of the cat retina (Nelson, 1980; Nelson et al., 1981; Nelson and Kolb, 1983).

Cb2 and cb6 have been demonstrated to give slow hyperpolarizing responses to light and to have large receptive fields with no sign of antagonistic surrounds (Nelson and Kolb, 1983). The HRP injected cb2 and cb6 cells can be examined in the electron microscope for synaptic connections. Cb2 has been shown to make superficial or basal junction with cone pedicles at some distance away from the synaptic ribbon complex. Cb6, on the other hand, has dendrites ending as both central elements below synaptic ribbons, but with a capping of horizontal cell processes between the bipolar endings and the synaptic ridge, and, in some instances, as basal junctions with the surface of the cone pedicles. Cb5 bipolars have been shown to give slow, depolarizing responses to light and an antagonistic surround can be elicited in the periphery of the narrow receptive field center (Nelson and Kolb, 1983). The dendritic contacts of cb5 with cone pedicles prove to be basal junctions ending close to the synaptic ribbon complex. The cb5 dendrites actually penetrate the cone pedicle to lie close to the synaptic ribbon but do so on either side of a centrally projecting bipolar dendrite belonging to another bipolar cell type. The synaptic contacts of the cb5 in the cat retina resemble those of the flat midget bipolar of the rhesus monkey (Figure 3). A fortuitously HRP stained, but not intracellularly recorded, cb3 bipolar of the cat has also been studied for synaptic connections. Its dendritic contacts with cones are fully invaginating: the dendrites end close to the synaptic ridge in the central position without any intervening cap of horizontal cell processes. Finally, the connections of cb1 are known from the Golgi-EM study (Boycott and Kolb, 1973) and serial section EM analysis (Kolb, 1979) although the intracellular physiology has not yet been recorded. Cb1 proves to have similar contacts with the cone pedicle as those of the cb5, in that the dendrites end on the base of the cone pedicle on either side of a central invaginating element.

All the cone bipolar cells of the cat retina that have been studied by electron microscopy appear to have direct synaptic output to ganglion cells, in contrast to the rod system where the rod bipolars do not have synapses with ganglion cells directly and use a variety of amacrine cells as interneurons (Kolb and Famiglietti, 1974). A detailed study concerning synaptology of the IPL such as performed on the cat retina has not yet been done on the rhesus monkey retina, but the same general principles concerning rod and cone bipolar wiring are thought to be in effect. For example, the AII amacrine, known to be integral to the rod pathway in cat retina is present in monkey and makes the same characteristic connections with rod bipolars and cone bipolars (Famiglietti and Kolb, 1975; Kolb, unpublished). Furthermore, Allen (1969), in his elegant serial section reconstructions of bipolar endings in the human retina, most of which were almost certainly midget cone bipolar axon terminals, showed that the majority of the bipolar synapses were to ganglion cell dendrites, just as in cat retina.

In cat IPL the cone bipolar synapses upon ganglion cell dendrites can take different forms. Most typically the synapses consist of a dyad of two postsynaptic profiles at the small ribbon in the cone bipolar terminal, one of which is a ganglion cell dendrite and the other an amacrine cell dendrite (Figure 6). Usually the synapse is wide-cleft with postsynaptic specialization on the ganglion or amacrine cell side of the membrane, and frequently the amacrine profile engages in a reciprocal synapse with the cone bipolar terminal (Figure 6). Where the ribbon synapses can be recognized to be from cbl bipolars the major synaptic specialization is between the cone bipolar and the ganglion cell dendrite, but the edge of a lobular appendage of the AII amacrine cell is sometimes involved (Famiglietti and Kolb, 1975) (Figure 7). Fairly common synapses observed in the neuropil of the IPL are monads between cone bipolar axon terminals and ganglion cell dendrites i.e. the ganglion cell is the only postsynaptic profile at the ribbon in the cone terminal (Figure 8), and sometimes the ribbon itself appears to be lacking (Figure 9). The conclusion to be drawn from the ultrastructural appearance of the cone bipolar to ganglion cell synapses in the cat retina, is that they are excitatory. Raviola and Raviola (1982), in fact, come to similar conclusions based on freeze-fracture appearances of synaptic specializations in the IPL of monkey and rabbit retinas.

GANGLION CELLS

Kuffler (1953) first described ganglion cells in the cat retina that responded with either ON or OFF centers and gave antagonistic responses in the surround region of their receptive fields. Later the commmonly recorded varieties of ganglion cell in the cat were classified on physiological criteria as X, Y (Enroth-Cugell and Robson, 1966) or W cells (Stone and Hoffman, 1972), brisk sustained or brisk transient (Cleland and Levick, 1974a), or sustained and transient (Fukuda and Stone, 1974; Ikeda and Wright, 1972). On morphological criteria cat ganglion cells have been classified as alpha, beta and gamma cells (Boycott and Wässle, 1974) or G1 to G23 (Kolb et al., 1981). Of this variety of classification schemes it is now accepted that the morphological types alpha, beta and gamma cells are the equivalent of concentrically organized Y, X and one type of W cell respectively.

The X cells of the cat retina are small-field concentric units equivalent to beta cells. They are most numerous and densely packed at the area centralis where they also have the smallest dendritic field sizes (Stone, 1965; Boycott and Wässle, 1974; Kolb et al., 1981). In addition beta cells project to the geniculo-striate (Wässle et al., 1981b; Leventhal et al., 1980; Leventhal, 1982) in a manner similar to monkey midget ganglion cell projections to the parvocellular geniculo-striate areas of the monkey visual system (Leventhal et al., 1981). It appears that the beta cells of the cat retina are analogous to, but as we shall see below, not exactly equivalent to, the midget ganglion cell system of the primate.

Nelson et al., (1978), by means of intracellular recordings of ganglion cells with the addition of dye injections to allow recorded cells to be visualized, confirmed for cat retina the original hypothesis of Gouras (1971) concerning the origin of receptive field center responses. Ganglion cells that have OFF center receptive fields, irrespective of their morphology of classification as X, Y or W cells (Enroth-Cugell and Robson, 1966; Stone and Hoffman, 1972), brisk sustained or brisk transient (Cleland and Levick, 1974a) have dendrites branching in neuropil of the IPL, called sublamina a (Famiglietti and Kolb, 1976) closest to the amacrine cells. Conversely, ganglion cells that give ON center responses have dendrites branching in lower IPL, called sublamina b (Famiglietti and Kolb, 1976) closest to the ganglion cell bodies. With the knowledge gained from the intracellular recordings it became evident that the two morphological groups of ganglion cells in the cat retina known as alpha and beta cells (Boycott and Wässle, 1974) occurred as paramorphic pairs across the entire retina (Famiglietti

Figures 6-9: Electron micrographs of cone bipolar synapses with ganglion and amacrine cells in the IPL of the cat retina. Figure 6: Ribbon synapses (small arrows) in the cone bipolar axon terminal (CB) point to two postsynaptic profiles, one of which is usually a ganglion (G) cell and the other an amacrine (A) cell dendrite. A slightly widened cleft and postsynaptic density characterize the synapses. Frequently the amacrine dendrite makes reciprocal synapses upon the cone bipolar axon terminal (large open arrow), X 43,000. Figure 7: A cone bipolar cell with its axon ending in sublamina a of the IPL (probably a cbl) makes a ribbon synapse to a ganglion cell dendrite (G). A tip of an AII lobular appendage is sometimes a second postsynaptic element, X 60,000. Figure 8: A ribbon synapse in a cone bipolar axon terminal (CB) lies above a single postsynaptic ganglion cell dendrite (G). This is a monad, X 64,500. Figure 9: Ribbonless monad synapse with a ganglion cell (G) postsynaptic to a cone bipolar (CB) axon terminal, X 43,000.

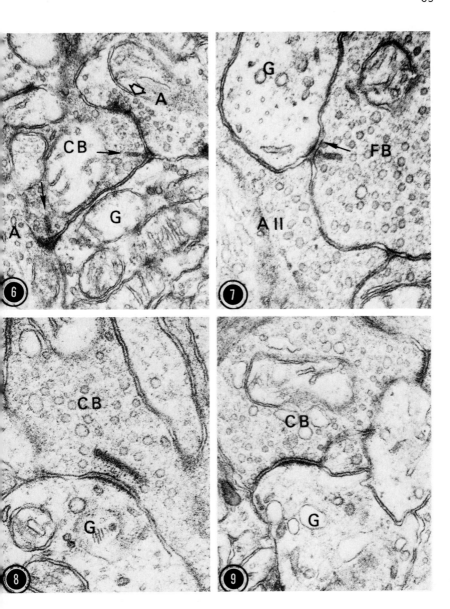

and Kolb, 1976; Wässle et al., 1981a and b). Both alpha and beta cells consisted of a types (OFF center) that branched in sublamina a, and b types (ON center) that branched in sublamina b. It was further thought that the ON and OFF center dichotomy of ganglion cells was intimately related to the type of cone bipolar input the pair of ganglion cells received (Famiglietti and Kolb, 1976) by analogy to the midget bipolar cell/midget ganglion cell situation in rhesus monkey retina.

Reconstructions from serial ultrathin sections of two small-field beta ganglion cells of the cat retina (Kolb, 1979) (Figure 10) has confirmed their cone bipolar cell relationships. The type a beta cell receives input only from cone bipolars that have axons restricted to sublamina a (cb1 and cb2) (Figure 10 and Figure 5). The type b beta cells, on the other hand, receive input only from cone bipolars that branch in sublamina b (cb5 and cb6). Similar findings for synaptic input to beta cells comes from the serial section reconstructions of Stevens et al. (1980) in cat retina. Beta a ganglion cells are known to give OFF center responses to irradiance of their receptive field center and beta b cell types are known to give ON center responses (Nelson et al., 1978; 1981; Nelson and Kolb, 1983). Synapses of the cone bipolar cells which are the major neuronal input to these ganglion cells are thought to be excitatory by both morphological and electrophysiological criteria (Kolb, 1979; Raviola and Raviola, 1982; Naka, 1976; Miller, 1980). Therefore, it appears that the center responses of the beta ganglion cells of the cat retina originate with the cone bipolar cells driving them.

Figure 11 summarizes the electrophysiological findings we have at present concerning the origin of the receptive field of beta ganglion cell types in the cat retina (Nelson and Kolb, 1983). The intracellular response of the cone photoreceptor in the cat is a slow hyperpolarization to light (Nelson, 1977). However, the cone bipolar cells postsynaptic to the cone photoreceptor can respond with either a hyperpolarization or a depolarization to light stimulation of their receptive field centers (Figure 11). Thus the original cone signal of an OFF center response, has been split into ON center (cb5) and OFF center (cb2, cb6) bipolar channels at the first synaptic level. OFF center beta cells are known to be driven by cb1 and cb2 bipolars. Of these only cb2 has so far been recorded from with intracellular techniques (Figure 11). Thus we know that at least one of the bipolar types driving beta OFF center ganglion cells are doing so through an excitatory (sign conserving) synapse, and the ganglion cell center response reflects the center response

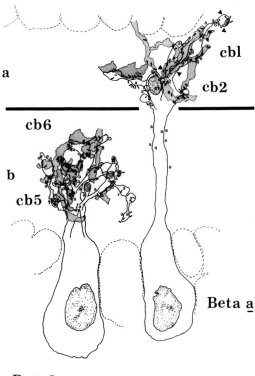

a

cbl

cb2

cb6

b

cb5

Beta a

Beta b

Figure 10: Drawing of two Beta ganglion cells that have been studied and reconstructed from serial EM sections, in the area centralis of the cat retina. Beta a branches in sublamina a and receives synaptic input primarily from cone bipolars (shaded profiles) of the type cbl and cb2. Arrowheads denote AII amacrine cell input and small a indicates unidentified amacrine synapses upon the apical dendrite and secondary dendritic appendages. The Beta b cell branches in neuropil close to its cell body in sublamina b. Its cone bipolar input (shaded profiles) cosists of cb5 and cb6 axon terminals although some minor proportion of amacrine cell input (a) also occurs. Modified from Kolb (1979).

of its input bipolar. For the ON center system, however, we see that both ON center (cb5) and an OFF center (cb6) cone bipolar has synaptic input to the ON center beta cell (Figure 11). Presumably, the cb5 bipolar with its ON center response to light is driving the ganglion cell with an excitatory (sign conserving) synapse, however, what of the cb6 which is known to have direct synapses with ON center beta cells?

Maguire et al. (1982) and Sterling (1983) have some evidence that a bipolar cell corresponding to cb6 takes up the inhibitory neurotransmitter glycine. They suggest, therefore, that cb6 input

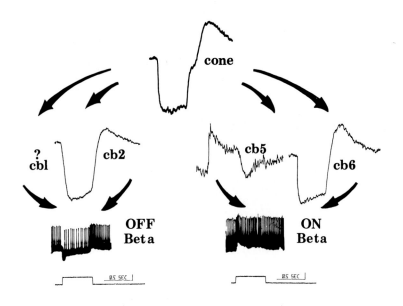

Figure 11: Intracellular responses of neurons involved in the major cone pathways to ganglion cells in the cat retina. The cone photoreceptor responds with a hyperpolarization (OFF) to central illumination. The cone bipolar cell (cb2) which has synapses upon OFF center Beta ganglion cell also responds with a hyperolarization (OFF) to light. The other cone bipolar synapsing upon OFF center Beta cells has not yet been intracellularly recorded (cbl?). The two cone bipolars that synapse upon ON center Beta cells are cb5 and cb6. Cb5 responds with a depolarization (ON) to central light illumination but the cb6 gives a hyperpolarizing (OFF) response. Arrows indicate the information flow from the cone through two pairs of bipolars to ON center and OFF center Beta ganglion cells.

to ON center ganglion cells will be inhibitory. They go on to speculate that glycinergic bipolar cells in both sublaminae are responsible for ON or OFF inhibition of the respective ganglion cells, rather than contributing to the receptive field center responses of the ganglion cells. This hypothesis would be attractive except that electrophysiological evidence suggests that OFF inhibition in ON center ganglion cells is GABA sensitive not glycine sensitive, and amacrine cell circuitry is considered responsible, (Miller, 1980; Ikeda and Sheardown, 1983). If the cb6 bipolar is to be considered important in the formation of the receptive field center of the ON center ganglion cell we will have to invoke a sign inverting synapse between cb6 and the ganglion cell. Ultrastructure and freeze-fracture studies argue that all bipolar to ganglion cell synapses are excitatory. Yet there is precedent for a bipolar cell in the cat IPL to make such sign inverting synapses, but to amacrine cells:

the rod bipolar cell is thought to make sign inverting synapses to at least one variety of amacrine cell (Nelson et al., 1976; Nelson, 1982; Kolb and Nelson, 1983).

AMACRINE CELLS IN THE CONE SYSTEM

The beta ganglion cells of the cat retina have been seen to have their major synaptic input from bipolar cells of either sub-lamina a or sublamina b (Figure 10) (Kolb, 1979; Stevens et al., 1980). However, it has also been noted that a considerable number of amacrine synapses impinge upon the dendrites and even on cell bodies of beta cells (Figure 10). The question is how might such amacrines be involved in the construction of the beta or X cell's concentric receptive field?

Two amacrine cell types of the cat retina, thought to play a role in the wiring of the beta cell receptive field, have been recorded from, marked with dye injection and indentified according to the Golgi classification scheme of Kolb et al., (1981). The A4 is a small-field amacrine cell with a compact, tufted dendritic tree branching in sublamina a, just above the a/b border (Figure 12A). The small spread of the dendritic tree and its intertwined dendrites have made this cell type amenable to serial section analysis by electron microscopy (Kolb, 1979). The findings of the EM analysis are depicted in Figure 12b. A4 receives synaptic input from, and makes reciprocal synapses with, cone bipolars that branch in S2 or sublamina a which are either or both the axon terminals of cb1 and cb2 (Figure 12B). The A4 amacrine also synapses upon dendrites of OFF center ganglion cells that branch in sublamina a. Some of these dendrites are characteristic of beta a type cells. Furthermore, the dendrites the A4 receive a large number of synapses from other unidentifiable amacrine cell types. The intracellular recordings of A4 indicate that it has an OFF center response to cone stimulating conditions, no surround antagonism but a very small receptive field (160μm) diameter (Kolb and Nelson, 1981). Interestingly, the receptive field of the A4 amacrine is considerably smaller than that of a cb2 which is providing some of its input (900um diameter). At present, of course, we have no way of knowing whether A4 might not more accurately reflect the receptive field size of a cb1 bipolar from which it receives input, for information concerning cb1's receptive field size is not yet available. If the A4 to ganglion cell synapse is sign conserving then the A4 should add to the exci-tatory receptive field center of the OFF center beta cell. If, on

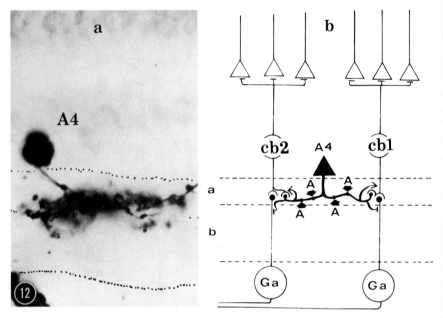

Figure 12: Golgi-impregnated appearance of an A4 amacrine cell in vertical section to show its narrow-field, tufted dendritic tree branching at the a/b border of the IPL. X 1,030. b) Summary diagram of the synaptic connections of the A4 amacrine cell as revealed by serial section EM. A4 is postsynaptic with reciprocal synapses to cb1 and cb2 bipolars and presynaptic to OFF center ganglion cells (Ga) in sublamina a. Unidentified amacrine cells (A) synapse upon the dendrites of A4.

the other hand, the A4 synapses are sign inverting one might propose that A4 is involved in ON inhibition of the OFF center ganglion cell. In any event, because of the small receptive field size of the A4 it seem intuitively more likely to be providing input to the receptive field center of the beta ganglion cells, than to the inhibitory surround.

Another amacrine cell type that is judged to be involved in the cone pathways to OFF center beta ganglion cells is A8 (Figure 13). This is a small-field, bistratified amacrine cell characterized by fine spidery dendrites ramifying in sublamina a and coarse, beaded dendrites in sublamina b (Figure 13A). The electron microscopic analysis of the HRP-stained and physiologically identified A8 indicates that the lower group of dendrites in sublamina b are post-synaptic to rod bipolar and cb6 axon terminals. There are recipro-cal synapses to the input cone bipolars (Figure 13B). The finer dendrites in sublamina a receive input from either or both cb1 and cb2 (Figure 13B) as well as from a number of unidentified amacrine cells. The A8 is presynaptic in sublamina a to OFF center beta

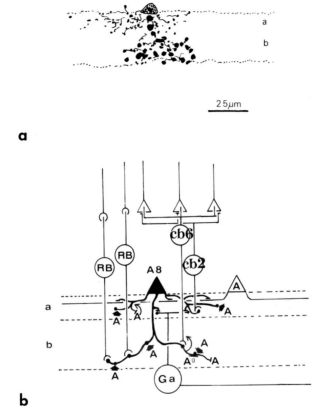

a

b

Figure 13: a) Camera lucida drawing of an A8 amacrine cell that has been stained with HRP after intracellular recording. In vertical section view the cell can be seen to have a narrow-field bistratified dendritic tree, with fine spidery dendrites proximal to its cell body and beaded dendrites in sublamina b. b) Summary drawing of the synaptic connections of A8 as revealed by serial section EM. The large beaded dendrites in sublamina b receive synapses from rod and cb6 cone bipolar axon terminals with reciprocal synapses to the cb6, in sublamina a, its fine dendrites are postsynaptic to cb2 axon terminal and presynaptic to OFF center ganglion cells (Ga) and a large radiate amacrine cell type. Amacrine synapses (A) are abundant on all parts of A8's dendritic tree. Scale bar=25 µm.

cells and to amacrine cell dendrites of extremely large diameter and radiate morphology, suggestive of an amacrine named A19 (Kolb et al., 1981). The intracellular recordings of A8 show that it is a hyperolarizing unit with a very pronounced OFF response. Stimulation with 677nm light designed to stimulate the cone system maximally, enhances the spikey OFF response while the 441nm light source, stimulating the rod system, eliminates the OFF response. An analysis of its receptive field shows that a strong depolarizing surround response can be elicited in this unit when the stimulus is displaced 500um from its receptive field center (Kolb and Nelson, 1981). In fact, the response characteristics of the A8 amacrine are very similar to the responses of an OFF center beta or X cell in the cat retina. It seems reasonable to suggest, therefore, that the A8 has direct excitatory synaptic input to the ganglion cells it is driving and provides both center and surround responses.

CONCENTRIC ORGANIZATION OF GANGLION CELLS

It was originally suggested that the surround of the concentric ganglion cells originated in the OPL (Dowling and Werblin, 1969; Dowling, 1970). In most submammalian species studied with intracellular techniques, it has been found that the bipolar cells have a concentric organization (Werblin and Dowling, 1969; Kaneko, 1970; Naka, 1976; Lasansky, 1978; Miller and Dacheux, 1976, Yazulla, 1976; Marchiafava and Weiler, 1980). The surround response of opposite polarity to the center response in the bipolar cell is thought to come from horizontal cells with their larger spatial characteristics, by means of either direct chemical synapses to bipolar cells (Dowling and Werblin, 1969; Kaneko, 1970; Naka, 1976) or through feedback to the photoreceptors (Toyoda, 1982, 1983). In the mammalian retina, though, the majority of bipolar cells do not appear to have antagonistic surrounds as part of their response characteristics (Nelson and Kolb, 1983). All the hyperpolarizing bipolar types, including the rod bipolar, cannot be induced to show any antagonistic surround. Their responses are very like those of horizontal cells of the cat (Nelson, 1977). The only bipolar cell in the cat retina to have a demonstrable surround is the depolarizing cone bipolar, cb5, but this surround appears to originate with the AII amacrine cell (Nelson, 1982). At scotopic light intensities where the AII amacrine is responding maximally, the cb5 has a response that mimics closely the AII amacrine. At photopic intensities were the cb5 is driven solely by the cone photoreceptor and where the AII amacrine is silent the antagonistic surround cannot be elicited. It is though that, under scoptopic conditions, the AII amacrine cell influences the cb5 cone bipolar by electrical (gap) junctions (Famiglietti and Kolb, 1975; Kolb and Nelson, 1983).

Even if it could be argued that surrounds have somehow not been recorded in cat bipolar cells due to the sensitivity of the preparation, Nelson (1977) has shown by measurements of space constants on

a large sample of horizontal cells of cat retina, that their receptive fields are too small to account for the spatial characteristics
of surrounds of even the smallest X cells of the area centralis. It
is, thus, thought more likely, that a major contribution to the
contruction of the surround of concentric ganglion cells in cat is
from amacrine cell pathways. In fact, two amacrine cell varieties,
namely AII and A8, known to have synaptic input to concentric ganglion cells, already have their own pre-wired concentric organization (Nelson et al., 1976; Kolb and Nelson 1981; Nelson 1982).

CONVERGENCE UPON HIGH ACUITY BETA (X) CELLS

Concentrically organized ganglion cell types of the cat retina
are arranged in regular, superimposed bi-level mosaics across the
whole retina (Wässle et al., 1981a,b). The cells have the smallest
dendritic field sizes at the area centralis and radiate out from the
central point with gradually expanding but essentially circular
dendritic fields. Each point on the retina is covered by at least
one OFF center cell and one ON center cell of the alpha and beta
type (Wässle et al., 1981a,b). The organization of the area centralis with densely packed, smallest-field beta cells and the
highest concentration of cone photoreceptors assures the lowest
convergence ratio of cones to ON center and OFF center X ganglion
cells. This organization is presumed to be the substrate for the
high acuity pathways of the cat.

It is not known whether in cat, as in monkey, the exact same
cones are connected by a bipolar cell innervating an ON center
ganglion cell and a neighboring bipolar innervating the partner OFF
center ganglion cell. However, the ratio of 30,000 cones (Steinberg
et al., 1973) to 4000 beta cells (Wässle et al., 1981b) per square
millimeter in the area centralis, equates to approximately 7 cones
per ganglion cell in this area of retina. This means that every ON
center/OFF center pair of ganglion cells is probably receiving input
from approximately 14 cones. Figure 14 shows a schematic of the
possible wiring of an ON and OFF center pair of beta ganglion cells
via their respective bipolar cells. It is assumed that cb1 and cb5
are the narrow-field high acuity bipolar cells of the cat retina
responsible for excitatory center mechanism to the ganglion cells.
Because we know that these narrow field bipolars contact between 4
and 8 cones in the area centralis (Boycott and Kolb, 1973), 14 cones
would be innervated by approximately 3 cone bipolars. The EM serial
section analysis of the central beta cells (Kolb, 1979) indicated

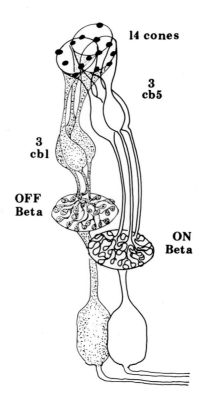

Figure 14: Schematic of the probable wiring of ON center and OFF center Beta cells of the area centralis of the cat's retina. There are approximately 14 cones converging on two Beta ganglion cells. Three cone bipolars of the narrowest-field type (cb1 and cb5) connect with the field of 14 cones to innervate each ganglion cell. OFF center cb1 bipolars have synaptic input to OFF center Beta cells while ON center cb5 bipolars have synaptic input to ON center Beta ganglion cells. Information from the same group of cones is fed through the parallel cone bipolar channels to parallel ON center and OFF center ganglion cell channels to the brain.

that only a very small number of narrow-field bipolar cell axons were providing the majority of the bipolar synapses to these beta cells, which is consistent with the small number innervating the available cones. It, therefore, seems likely that the same group of cones are wired to both ON center and OFF center beta ganglion cells through about three cone bipolars per ganglion cell (Figure 14). Thus, in all likelihood, in the cat retina, identical visual space looked at by the same photoreceptors is being channeled into the parallel ON center and OFF center ganglion cell pathways to the higher visual centers.

CONCLUSIONS AND COMPARISONS BETWEEN THE CONE PATHWAYS OF CAT AND
MONKEY RETINAS

We have learned much concerning the synaptic circuitry underlying high acuity pathways of the cat retina from the combination of
anatomical and physiological approaches. This type of analysis has
not yet been possible in the monkey retina and so at present we must
draw conclusions concerning the wiring of the monkey ganglion cells
receptive fields from the findings in the cat. We believe that the
basic pattern of parallel ON center and OFF center channels through
the monkey retina originate, as with the cat, by a dual cone bipolar
system segregating input to parallel ganglion cell varieties branching at the two levels of the neuropil of the IPL. We further
conclude that the receptive field center of the parallel ganglion
cell channels are provided by the excitatory cone bipolar input, but
the wiring of the antagonistic surround is provided by amacrine cell
pathways. However, it is quite clear that the monkey retina with
its much higher acuity visual system than the cat has finely tuned
the construction of the visual message by employing the single cone
connections of the midget bipolar and midget ganglion cell systems.
Because of the insufficient cone photoreceptor density and packing
compared with the primate retina, and the bipolars having convergent
photoreceptor input, the beta cells of the cat retina have a coarser
tuning than midget ganglion cells of the primate retina.

Comparisons of the morphology of the different types of ganglion cells in the monkey (Polyak, 1941; Kolb, unpublished) and cat
retina (Boycott and Wässle, 1974; Kolb et al., 1981) indicate that
the monkey retina has paramorphic pairs of small-field ganglion
cells, called parasol cells, which are similar in appearance to the
beta ganglion cells of cat, in addition to its unique midget ganglion cells. Table I shows the probable equivalent ganglion cells
in cat and monkey retinas. As can be seen, many of the same types
of cells are found in both species, including cells equivalent to
alpha and beta cells of the cat, but clearly the midget ganglion
cells are the ultimate refinements of the geniculo-striate system in
primates, and have developed as a parallel system to that of the
still existent beta cell system.

It is interesting that in the foveal region of the monkey
retina, the size of the dendritic trees of the parasol ganglion
cells, so similar to cat beta cells, is three or four times that of
the midget ganglion cell (Polyak, 1941), suggesting input from a
group of convergent bipolar cells. Polyak (1941) suggested that

TABLE I

SIMILAR GANGLION CELLS IN CAT AND RHESUS MONKEY RETINAS

CAT	MONKEY
–	midget $\underline{a}$
–	midget $\underline{b}$
beta $\underline{a}$	parasol $\underline{a}$
beta $\underline{b}$	parasol $\underline{b}$
alpha $\underline{a}$	giant (parasol) $\underline{a}$
alpha $\underline{a}$	giant (parasol) $\underline{b}$
G17, G14, G15	garland
G5, G4, G18	small diffuse
–	biplexiform (Mariani, 1982)

midget bipolar cells as well as two varieties of diffuse cone bipolar cell would converge on the parasol ganglion cells of central retina. This brings us back to the relationship between the cone bipolar cells of the monkey and cat. Table II indicates the possible equivalent bipolar cells in the two species. The cells are compared on morphological similarities such as branching levels of their axons in the IPL and the nature of their dendritic contacts with cone pedicles. The diffuse cone bipolars of monkey and the wide-field bipolars of cat are clearly comparable. The midget bipolars are considered to be the equivalent of cat narrow-field cb1 and cb5, respectively, for three reasons. Firstly, in both species their axon terminals are very strictly related to the sublaminae of the IPL and their compact arrangement allows maximum coverage of the dendritic tree of the ganglion cell with which they synapse in both cases. Secondly, the midget bipolars are thought to have a minor contribution of their synaptic output to parasol ganglion cells which are equivalent to cat beta cells. Thirdly, midget bipolars can become two or three headed in peripheral primate retina (Polyak, 1941; Kolb, unpublished), giving them a polysynaptic morphology very similar to cb1 or cb5 of cat area centralis. In fact, in the owl monkey where the fovea is less well developed and the retina has a greater proportion of rods more like the cat retina, the midget bipolars are almost all polysynaptic (Ogden, 1974).

It now seems likely that the midget bipolars of the rhesus monkey retina are only related to the red and green cones. The blue cones may be contacted by a unique type of bipolar (the single-cone-contacting, non-midget bipolar, Mariani, 1982), which substitutes for the midget system. The other diffuse varieties of cone bipolars in rhesus are presumed to contact all three cone types. Because blue cones are well developed in the cat retina it might be that cb6 is the equivalent of the unique polysynaptic blue cone bipolar of

TABLE II

SIMILAR BIPOLAR CELLS IN CAT AND RHESUS MONKEY RETINAS

CAT	MONKEY
cb1:semi-invag.	midget flat:semi-invag
cb5:semi-invag.	midget invag:invag.
cb2:flat	diffuse flat:flat
cb3:invag.	diffuse invaginating:invag.
cb4:?	bistratified:flat (Mariani,1982)
cb6:	single-cone, non-midget (Mariani,1982):
large invag.	large invag.
cb7:?	—
cb8:?	—

the monkey retina. At present these comparisons between cat and monkey retinas are still in the realms of speculation and future research will have to identify the spectral cone types in both species in order to further our understanding of their bipolar and ganglion cell connections.

ACKNOWLEDGEMENTS

I thank Dr. Ralph Nelson for allowing me to reproduce some of his physiological data. Supported by Grant EY 03323 from the National Eye Institute.

REFERENCES

Allen, R.A. (1969). The retinal bipolar cells and their synapses in the inner plexiform layer. In The retina: morphology, function and clinical characteristics. (eds. Straatsma, B.R., Hall, M.O., Allen, R.A. and Crescitelli, F.) pp. 101-143. Forum in Medical Sciences. No. 8 Berkeley: University of California Press.

Boycott, B.B. and Dowling, J.E. (1969). Organization of the primate retina: light microscopy. Phil. Trans. R. Soc. (Lond), B, 255: 109-184.

Boycott, B.B. and Kolb, H. (1973). The connections between the bipolar cells and photoreceptors in the retina of the domestic cat. J. Comp. Neur., 148: 91-114.

Boycott, B.B. and Wässle, H. (1974). The morphological types of ganglion cells of the domestic cat's retina. J. Physiol. (Lond), 240: 397-419.

Cajal, S.R. (1933). Die Retina der Wirbeltiere. Wiesbaden: Bergmann; Trans. Thorpe, S.A. and Glickstein, M. (1972). The Structure of the Retina. Thomas, Springfield.

Cleland, B.G. and Levick, W.R. (1974a). Brisk and sluggish concentrically organized ganglion cells in the cat's retina. J. Physiol. (Lond.), 240: 421-456.

Dowling, J.E. (1970). Organization of vertebrate retinas. Invest. Ophthal., 9: 655-680.

Dowling, J.E. and Werblin, F.S. (1969). Organization of the retina of the mudpuppy, Necturus maculosus. I. Synaptic structure. J. Neurophysiol., 32: 315-338.

Enroth-Cugell, C. and Robson, J.G. (1966). The contrast sensitivity of retinal ganglion cells of the cat. J. Physiol. (Lond.), 187: 517-552.

Famiglietti, E.V. and Kolb, H. (1975). A bistratified amacrine cell and synaptic circuitry in the inner plexiform layer of the retina. Brain Res. 84: 293-300.

Famiglietti, E.V. and Kolb, H. (1976). Structural basis for 'ON' and 'OFF'-center responses in retinal ganglion cells. Science 194: 193-195.

Fukuda, Y. and Stone, J. (1974). Retinal distribution and central projections of Y-, X-, and W-cells of the cat's retina. J. Neurophysiol., 37: 749-772.

Gouras, P. (1971). The function of the midget cell system in primate color vision. Vision Res. Suppl., 3: 397-410.

Ikeda, H. and Wright, M.J. (1972). Differential effects on refractive errors and receptive field organization of central and peripheral ganglion cells. Vision Res., 12: 1465-1476.

Ikeda, H. and Sheardown, M. (1983). Functional transmitters at retinal ganglion cells in the cat. Vision Res., 23: 1161-1174.

Kaneko, A. (1970). Physiological and morphological identification of horizontal, bipolar and amacrine cells in goldfish retina. J. Physiol. (Lond), 207: 623-633.

Kolb, H., Boycott, B.B. and Dowling, J.E. (1969). A second type of midget bipolar cell in the primate retina. Appendix. Phil Trans. R. Soc. (Lond.), B. 255: 177-184.

Kolb, H. (1970). Organization of the outer plexiform layer of the primate retina: electron microscopy of Golgi-impregnated cells. Phil. Trans. R. Soc. (Lond.), B, 258: 261-283.

Kolb, H. and Famiglietti, E.V. (1974). Rod and cone bipolar connections in the inner plexiform layer of the cat retina. Science 186: 47-49.

Kolb, H. (1979). The inner plexiform layer in the retina of the cat: electron microscope observations. J. Neurocytol., 8: 295-329.

Kolb, H. and Nelson, R. (1981). Three amacrine cells of the cat retina: morphology and intracellular responses. ARVO. Invest. Ophthal. Vis. Sci., Suppl., 20: p. 184.

Kolb, H., Nelson, R. and Mariani, A. (1981). Amacrine cells, bipolar cells and ganglion cells of the cat retina: a Golgi study. Vision Res., 21: 1081-1114.

Kolb, H. and Nelson, R. (1983). Rod pathways in the retina of the cat. Vision Res., 23:301-312.

Kuffler, S.W. (1953). Discharge patterns and functional organization of mammalian retina. J. Neurophysiol., 16: 47-68.

Lasansky, A. (1978). Contacts between receptors and electrophysiologically identified neurones in the retina of the larval Tiger Salamander. J. Physiol. (Lond), 285: 531-542.

Leventhal, A.G., Keens, J. and Türk, I. (1980). The afferent ganglion cells and cortical projections of the retinal recipient zone (RRZ) of the cat's 'Pulvinar complex'. J. Comp. Neur., 194: 535-554.

Leventhal, A.G., Rodieck, R.W. and Dreher, B. (1981). Retinal ganglion cell classes in old world monkeys: morphology and central projections. Science 213: 1139-1142.

Leventhal, A.G. (1982). Morphology and distribution of retinal ganglion cells projecting to different layers of the dorsal lateral geniculate nucleus in normal and siamese cats. J. Neurosci., 2: 1024-1042.

Maguire, B.A., Stevens, J.K. and Sterling, P. (1982). "Push-pull" microcircuitry of the beta (X) ganglion cell in light adaptation. ARVO. Invest. Ophthal. Vis. Sci., Suppl. 22, p. 82.

Marchiafava, P.L. and Weiler, R. (1980). Intracellular analysis and structural correlates of the organization of inputs to ganglion cells in the retina of the turtle. Proc. R. Soc. (Lond.) B, 208: 103-113.

Mariani, A.P. (1981). A diffuse, invaginating cone bipolar cell in primate retina. J. Comp. Neur. 197: 661-671.

Mariani, A.P. (1982). Newly identified bipolar cells in monkey retina. ARVO. Invest. Ophthal. Vis. Sci. Suppl. 22, p. 247.

Marr, D. (1974). The computation of lightness by the primate retina. Vision Res. 14: 1377-1388.

Miller, R.F. (1980). The neuronal basis of ganglion-cell receptive-field organization and the physiology of amacrine cells. In Neuronal Interactions in the Vertebrate Retina. Neurosciences fourth study program, 1979 (Eds. Schmitt, F.O. and Worden, F.G.) MIT Press, Cambridge, MA and London, England.

Miller, R.F. and Dacheux, R.F. (1976). Synaptic organization and ionic basis on On and Off channels in mudpuppy retina. I. Intracellular analysis of chloride-sensitive electrogenic properties of receptors, horizontal cells, bipolar cells and amacrine cells. J. Gen. Physiol. 67: 639-659.

Naka, K-I. (1976). Neuronal circuitry in the cat fish retina. Invest. Ophthal., 15: 926-935.

Nelson, R. (1977). Cat cones have rod input: a comparison of the response properties of cones and horizontal cell bodies in the retina of the cat. J. Comp. Neur., 172: 109-135.

Nelson, R. (1980). Functional stratification of cone bipolar axons in the cat retina. ARVO. Invest. Ophthal. Vis. Sci., Suppl., p. 130.

Nelson, R. (1982). AII amacrine cells quicken time course of rod signals in the cat retina. J. Neurophysiol. 47: 928-947.

Nelson, R., Famiglietti, E.V. and Kolb, H. (1978). Intracellular staining reveals different levels of stratification for on-center and off-center ganglion cells in the cat retina. J. Neurophysiol., 41:472-483.

Nelson, R., Kolb, H., Famiglietti, E.V. and Gouras, P. (1976). Neural responses in rod and cone systems of the cat retina: Intracellular staining reveals different levels of stratification for on-center and off-center ganglion cells in the cat retina. J. Neurophysiol. 41: 472-483.

Nelson, R., Kolb, H., Robinson, M.M. and Mariani, A.P. (1981). Neural activity of the cat retina: cone pathways to ganglion cells. Vision Res. 21: 1527-1536.

Nelson, R. and Kolb, H. (1983). Synaptic patterns and response properties of bipolar and ganglion cells in the cat retina. Vision Res., 23: 1183-1195.

Ogden, T.E. (1974). The morphology of retinal neurons of the owl monkey, Aotes. J. Comp. Neur., 153: 399-428.

Polyak, S.L. (1941). The Retina. Univ. of Chicago Press.

Raviola, E. and Raviola, G. (1982). Structure of the synaptic membranes in the inner plexiform layer of the retina. A freeze-fracture study in monkeys and rabbits. J. Comp. Neur., 209: 233-248.

Steinberg, R.H., Reid, M. and Lacey, P.L. (1973). The distribution of rods and cones in the retina of the cat (Felis domesticus). J. Comp. Neur., 148: 229-248.

Sterling, P. (1983). Microcircuitry of the cat retina. Ann. Rev. in Neurosci., 6: 149-183.

Stevens, J.K., McGuire, B.A. and Sterling, P. (1980). Toward a functional architecture of the retina: serial reconstruction of adjacent ganglion cels. Science 207: 317-319.

Stone, J. (1965). A quantitative analysis of the distribution of ganglion cells in the cat's retina: J. Comp. Neur. 124: 337-352.

Stone, LJ. and Hoffmann, K.P. (1972). Very slow-conduction ganglion cells in the cat's retina: a major new functional type? Brain Res., 43: 610-616.

Toyoda, J-I. and Kujiraoka, T. (1982). Analysis of bipolar cell respones elicited by polarization of horizontal cells. J. Gen. Physiol. 79: 131-145.

Toyoda, J-I. and Fugimoto, M. (1983). Analyses of neural mechanisms mediating the effect of horizontal cells polarization. Vision Res., 23: 1143-1150.

Wässle, H., Peichl, L. and Boycott, B.B. (1981a). Morphology and topography of on- and off- alpha cells in the cat retina. Proc. R. Soc. (Lond.), B, 212: 157-175.

Wässle, H., Boycott, B.B. and Illing, R.-B. (1981b). Morphology and mosaic of on- and off- beta cells in the cat retina and some functional considerations. Proc. R. Soc. (Lond.), B, 212: 177-195.

Werblin, F.S. and Dowling, J.E. (1969). Organization of the retina of the mdpuppy, Necturus maculosus. II. Intracellular recording. J. Neurophysiol., 32: 339-355.

Yazulla, S. (1976). Cone input to bipolar cells in the turtle retina. Vision Res., 16: 737-744.

Structure, Development and Visual Acuity in the Goldfish Retina

W.K. Stell and J-H. Kock

The retina is a complex instrument for detecting and analyzing the form, color, brightness and movement of visual stimuli. The first stage comprises the outer segments of photoreceptor cells, an array of detectors analogous in part to the array of silver halide crystals in a photographic emulsion. At each successive stage, however, the initial pointillistic array of picture elements is modified, distorted, almost beyond recognition. This process begins within the photoreceptors themselves, which are coupled electrically by means of gap junctions to form networks of homologous elements. It continues in the outer synaptic layer, where bipolar cells integrate photoreceptor inputs to varying degrees, differentiate between local photoreceptor inputs and global or adaptive horizontal cell inputs, and perform sign-conserving or sign-inverting operations related to positive and negative contrast detection. It attains its apotheosis, for the retina at least, in the inner synaptic layer, where there are so many structural elements, transmitters and visual functions that today we are at a complete loss to understand it. Suffice to say that the inner synaptic layer is the site of numerous spatial and temporal, linear-to-nonlinear transformations, with which my respected colleague and friend Ken Naka has been particularly concerned. Anatomically the visual pathways are also impressive, not only for their increasing complexity, but also for the steady increase in dendritic tree size along the path from receptor to brain.

Spatial acuity, the ability to resolve fine details of image structure, is generally understood to be limited by neural rather than optical factors (e.g. Easter et al., 1977). Considering the prominence of anatomical convergence and functional integration in the visual pathways (even of man with his renowned "private pathway" of cone-related midget cells), it is difficult sometimes to see clearly the basis for visual acuity in retinal circuitry. Lower vertebrates are useful for resolving such problems, because their simple behavior and hardy physiology make them accessible to evaluation at many levels of organization. Goldfish in particular is advantageous because it has rods, cones and color vision; its retinal structure is exceptionally well known; and its rod-related retinal circuitry changes constantly throughout life, presenting the opportunity for studying the adaptation of visual behavior to developmental alterations of neural organization.

In this paper we will discuss the synaptic interconnections of photoreceptor and bipolar cells in goldfish and other teleosts. We will describe changes in photoreceptor-bipolar cell interconnections observed during retinal growth. We will consider how the structure of photoreceptor-bipolar cell synapses may reveal fundamental rules of photoreceptor synaptogenesis and bipolar cell function. Finally, we will attempt to relate these facts of retinal synaptic structure and development to visual acuity and its development.

RETINAL STRUCTURE IN GOLDFISH

Photoreceptors. The goldfish retina contains rods and cones, in proportions that range from 100% cones at hatching to as little as 5% in large adults (Johns, 1982). The cones are pleiomorphic, with distinctive structural types containing distinctive spectral classes of visual pigments (Scholes, 1975; Marc & Sperling, 1976; Stell & Harosi, 1976). "Red-sensitive" (R; λ max ~ 620 nm) "green-sensitive" (G; λmax ~ 533 nm), and "blue-sensitive" (B; λmax 453 nm) cones are present, in the approximate proportions 0.45R: 0.35G: 0.20B (Stell, 1980). The absolute density of all cones per unit retinal area varies with retinal region by no more than a factor of two, and the proportions of cones of different types are the same in all regions (Marc & Sterling, 1976). The cones are arranged in an irregular square to rhombic mosaic, in which members of each of the major types are quasi-regularly arranged for near-maximum separation (Figure 1). The intercone distance for goldfish cones of a given chromatic type is, therefore, the average intercone distance divided by the proportional factor for that type; intercone distance for R cones is about 1.4 times, for G cones about 1.8 times, and for B cones about 2.4 times the average for all cones. The situation is similar in primates (Marc & Sperling, 1977).

Photoreceptor properties that may influence acuity include not only spatial separation (distribution) but also low-resistance junc-

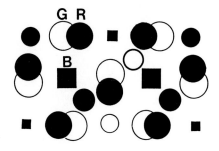

Figure 1. Schematic summary of spatial distributions of goldfish cones. Large paired circles represent unequal double cones (R = red-sensitive long double; G = green-sensitive short double), arranged in square units. Large squares represent short single cones (B). Long single cones are represented as circles of intermediate size (dark = R; light = G). Miniature single cones of each chromatic type are represented by the smallest symbols of each type. Average spatial distribution parameters for cones of each chromatic type are:

Type	Cones/mm^2 x 10^3	**Linear separation (μm)
B	2.7	20
G	4.8	14
R	6.5	12
Total	14	8.5

*Data for 11 cm (S.L.) fish; Stell & Harosi (1976).
**Approximately equal to angular substense (min.), assuming 60 μm/deg. in 11 cm fish; see e.g. Easter et al. (1977).

tions and interreceptor synapses. Thin-section studies in carp (Witkovsky, Shakib & Ripps, 1974) and freeze-fracture studies in goldfish (Nagy, Stell & Lightfoot, 1983) leave no doubt that gold-fish rods are coupled extensively through low resistance gap junc-tions, and suggest that some goldfish cones as well may be electri-cally coupled. One may expect, therefore, that the receptive field of goldfish cones is substantially larger than either the diameter of the cone itself or the distance between cones. While it has not been possible to measure receptive fields of goldfish cones, an upper limit may be estimated from measurements on the pike-perch, in which the diameter of cone receptive fields is about 100 μm (Burkhardt, 1977). The receptive fields of turtle cones, which are known to be coupled specifically to other cones of the same type, are also about 100 μm in diameter (Baylor et al, 1971; Baylor & Hodgkin, 1973). The spatial sensitivity function of goldfish cones, then, may also be bell-shaped with a half-width of 100 μm. The extent of summation among goldfish rods is even more difficult to estimate. In the snapping turtle, Chelydra, rod receptive fields are about 400 μm in diameter. Goldfish rod fields may be far smal-

;h rods are very much smaller and closer
ı lack their long telodendria (Nagy, et
, 1980). It is clear that electrical
:ocurrents in a cluster of cells and
:ontally, must also reduce resolution
t is not clear that there is any
resolution imposed by photoreceptor
_roximal retinal circuitry on the

_aily extending basal processes or telodendrons have
.. observed on photoreceptors in Golgi silver-chromate preparations of retinas from many species (Cohen, 1972). Lasansky (1971)
showed that some of the cone basal processes in a turtle ascend into
the synaptic cavities (invaginations) of other cones near by.
Scholes (1976) made the important discovery that in a cyprinid fish,
the rudd, the invaginating cone-cone interconnections are color-
coded: G cones into R cones, R cones into G cones, and B cones into
G cones. Lockhart and Stell (1979; see also Stell, 1980) found
goldfish to resemble rudd, with the addition of R and G cone telodendrons invaginating into B cones. The pattern of color-coding
suggests that invaginating telodendronal pathways may sharpen color
discrimination or contrast (Stell, 1980) over distances on the order
of 25 μm (radius from cone of origin).

Bipolar Cells. Teleostean bipolar cells comprise two classes:
pure cone and mixed rod-cone (Scholes, 1975; Stell, 1980); there are
no bipolars that receive from rods only, as in mammals (e.g. Kolb,
1970). Among the mixed rod-cone bipolars (Ishida et al., 1980),
dendritic tree diameter varies directly and linearly with number of
cones contacted (figure 2A) but it is unrelated to either number of
rods contacted (figure 2B) or ratio of rods:cones contacted (figure
2C).

Not only do all goldfish rod bipolars receive from cones as
well; but also those cones always include at least the red-sensitive
ones (Ishida et al, 1980). Even though the mechanism (kinetics and
transmitters) of rod- and cone-to-bipolar synaptic transmission
appear to differ, within the physiological range of membrane potentials the mixed bipolars respond to illumination of rods and cones
with changes of the same sign (Saito, Kondo & Toyoda, 1978, 1979).
One would expect therefore that rod and R-cone signals are additive
or synergistic upon the mixed bipolars, as suggested by behavioral
experiments (Powers & Easter, 1978), and that they might be equivalent at subsequent stages of visual processing such as ganglion

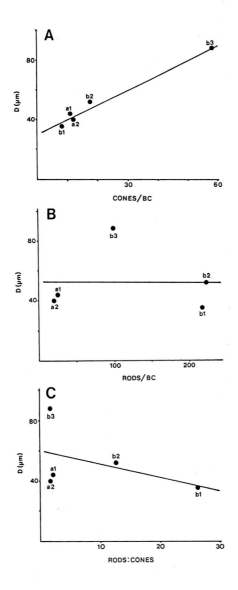

Figure 2. Graphs of dendritic tree diameters (D) of goldfish mixed rod-cone bipolar cells (types a1, a2, b1, b2, b3) against various photoreceptor parameters. Dendritic spread is strongly correlated with number of cones contacted (A), as expected since contacts are made with all cones of selected type within dendritic field, but poorly correlated with number of rods contacted (B) or ratio of rods contacted to cones contacted (C). Correlation coefficients (r) for linear regression functions are 0.99 (A), 0.51 (B) and 0.45 (C). Data from Ishida et al. (1980), Tables 1 & 2, p. 321.

cells (Beauchamp & Daw, 1972; Raynauld, 1972). The bipolar cells whose acuity (in a strictly geometrical sense) appears to be highest are the type b1 mixed bipolars, whose elliptical dendritic trees measure about 30 x 40 μm, on average; their dendrites contact all the rods and R cones within their field and overlap little with the dendrites of neighbouring b1 bipolars (Ishida et al, 1980). This places the minimum center–center separation of bipolars in the range of 35 μm in 11 cm fish.

Several peculiarities of the various types of mixed bipolar cells are worthy of note. First is that while all contact both rods and cones, the proportions of rod and cone contacts vary widely (Ishida et al, 1980). Electron microscopic studies, furthermore, reveal variations in dendritic connectivity with rods that suggest important functional differentiations and synaptogenetic mechanisms. Nine rod synapses in an 11 cm goldfish were sectioned serially for electron microscopy and reconstructed with computer assistance (Shantz & McCann, 1978; Stell & Lightfoot, 1979). Computer-estimated areas of specialized contact between rods and bipolar cell dendrites may be taken as a measure of relative functional influence of the rods upon the bipolars; taking these measured values into account, our data (Table 1) suggest that the weighting of rod input to different bipolar cell types may vary over nearly three orders of magnitude (Lightfoot et al, 1977; Stell & Lightfoot, 1979).

A second interesting point is that the shapes of the dendritic arborizations of the mixed bipolars are type-specific, varying regularly from type to type; all are more or less elliptical in horizontal projection, but with ratios of maximum:minimum diameter that represent them as nearly circular (a2: 1.20; b2: 1.16), slightly compressed (b1: 1.35; b3: 1.47), to markedly flattened (a1: 2.80). In all cases the major diameters are oriented normal to retinal meridians (Ishida et al, 1980). This observation raises the possibility of "orientation bias" in the acuity-related functional properties of these cells, as Levick and Thibos (1982) have reported

TABLE 1

BIPOLAR CELL TYPE	PHOTORECEPTORS PER BIPOLAR			ROD–BIPOLAR SYNAPTIC AREA $\mu m^2 x 10^{-3}$ per bipolar	ROD–BIPOLAR SYNAPTIC AREA (μm^2/bipolar)
	R CONES	G CONES	RODS		
b1	8.3	0	218	638	139.0
b2	9.7	8.0	223	137	30.6
b3	35.0	22.5	100	18	1.8
a1	11.4	0	25	52	1.3
a2	7.3	4.8	20	20	0.4

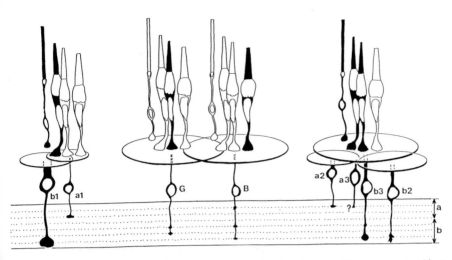

Figure 3. Diagram of known types of bipolar cells in goldfish retina. Mixed rod-cone bipolars are represented by 3 types (a1, a2, a3) that respond to focal illuminaton by hyperpolarization and terminate in the distal sublamina (a) of the inner synaptic layer, and by 3 types (b1, b2, b3) that respond to focal illumination by depolarization and terminate in the proximal sublamina (b) of the inner synaptic layer; one subtype each (a1, b1) contacts only R cones whereas two subtypes each (a2, a3, b2, b3) contact both R & G cones. Pure cone bipolars are represented by two types with much larger dendritic fields than the mixed bipolars, one specific for G cones and cone for B cones, with uncertain destinations in the inner synaptic layer. Other pure cone bipolars probably exist (cf. Scholes, 1975) but have not yet been described in goldfish. Redrawn and modified from Stell (1980).

for ganglion cells in the cat.

Third, there is the interesting functional division of bipolar cells into two types, center-hyperpolarizing (OFF) and center-depolarizing (ON). The levels of terminal arborization of bipolar cell axons in the inner plexiform layer (IPL) are related to function: in carp, as in the cat (Famiglietti & Kolb, 1976), hypolarizing bipolars end in the distal part, or sublamina a, of the IPL whereas depolarizing bipolars end in the proximal part, or sublamina b, of the IPL (Famiglietti et al., 1977). The type a mixed bipolars, therefore, are functionally center hypolarizing (inactivated by illumination), whereas the type b mixed bipolars are functional center-depolarizing (activated by illumination). The type b1 and b2 bipolars, whose inputs are rod-rich (rods:cones = 26.3 and 12.6), appear to be the best candidates for the spatial acuity-limiting bipolar cell channels at threshold for increment detection. In contrast, the type a1 and a2 bipolars, whose inputs are rod-poor (rods:cones = 2.2 and 1.7), appear to be corresponding channels for decrement detection. This dichotomy makes sense, since rods can be expected to be the best detectors of light at threshold (in the dark) whereas cones can be expected to detect decrements most readily (Normann & Werblin, 1974; Baylor & Fettiplace, 1977). Within classes a and b there are further matched pairs - a1 and b1 being most sensitive to long wavelengths, a2 and b2 having broader sensitivities extending also into middle wavelengths. It appears likely (Stell, 1979) that these are "color-opponent" (Kaneko, 1973) or "double-color-opponent" (Kaneko & Tachibana, 1981) bipolars as described in carp. It is probably significant that the least radially symmetric mixed bipolar type a1, is a rod-poor, R-cone-only, center-hyperpolarizing type, but that significance is not clear at present.

A sixth mixed rod-cone bipolar cell type is probably present in goldfish. In earlier studies (Stell, 1976) we observed slender dendrites, centrally placed, in triads of R-cone ribbon synapses. Now the homologous cell has been identified in carp retina. Saito et al. (1983) have recorded intracellularly from a hyperpolarizing bipolar and marked it with HRP for further study. Electron microscopy showed this cell's dendrites to end near the synaptic ridge in rods and G cones as well as in the center of R-cone triads. Its center-hyperpolarizing response is anticipated from the finding of Nagy et al. (1983) that the membranes of the presumed bipolar cell dendrites in R-cone triads are decorated with E-face particles, that is, their dendrites are postsynaptic in presumed sign-conserving ("excitatory") synapses. While Saito and colleagues did not mention the level of termination of their OFF-bipolar in the inner synaptic layer, we may assume that it follows the same rule as other carp bipolars and ends in sublamina a. We feel justified, therefore, in naming this cell in carp, and its equivalent in gold-fish, type a3, even though its junctional ultrastructure differs from that of types a1 and a2, from which Saito and colleagues appear not to have recorded (and marked).

Horizontal Cells. Teleostean horizontal cells were probably the first retinal cells to be studied by intracellular recording (Svaetichin, 1953) and are arguably the best understood of any retinal cells. The subject has been reviewed exhaustively in a recent volume commemorating Svaetichin's seminal discovery (Drujan & Laufer, 1982), and an article on goldfish has appeared in that volume (Stell, Kretz & Lightfoot, 1982). Since the role of horizontal cells in spatial acuity appears to be rather limited, compared to its roles in chromatic and temporal processing, a cursory summary will suffice here.

Teleostean horizontal cells contact either rods or cones, never both, in all species examined (Cajal, 1892; Stell, 1967; Parthe, 1982; Wagner, 1978; Van Haesendonck & Missotten, 1979). The rod horizontal cells are of a single type, whereas the cone horizontal cells generally comprise two or more types differing in cone connectivity. With the exception of a brief report by Wagner and Speck (1982), detailed examination of functionally identified horizontal cells in carp and goldfish confirms the model outlined by Stell and Lightfoot (1975): (1) Each of three cone horizontal cell types receives primarily (or exclusively) from one of the three cone types. (2) Each of these cone-to-horizontal cell synapses is sign-conserving; light causes both cones and horizontal cells to hyperpolarize. (3) Cone horizontal cells act in part to impose new chromatic properties upon one another, because they are functionally (chromatically) polarized; R-cone-dominated horizontal cells influence G-cone-dominated horizontal cells, which in turn influence B-cone-dominated horizontal cells. (4) This interaction is chromatically opponent; the result is a red-opponent (R-depolarizing) system in the G-cone-dominated horizontal cell and a green-opponent (G-depolarizing) system in the B-cone-dominated horizontal cell. (5) Cone horizontal cell interactions are mediated, at least in part, by "feedback" synapses of horizontal cells upon cones, which may be gaba-ergic in the case of R-cone-dominated (CH1, external, or L-type) horizontal cells. (6) Horizontal cells of like type are coupled electrically by gap junctions to form a leaky functional syncytium, called by Naka "S-space". (7) Horizontal cell coupling, combined with either "feedback" or "feedforward" synapses, allows the input to (and output from) bipolar cells to reflect the average brightness and chromaticity of illumination over a wide surrounding area.

Some Acuity-Related Consequences of Horizontal Cell Function. Consequences of horizontal cell activity are numerous and by no means yet comprehensively appreciated. We will focus upon those that are most relevant to spatial acuity, first in an achromatic and then in a chromatic environment.

In the dark, and in the absence of horizontal cell function, a bipolar cell responds to the image of a small object (spot of light) entering the receptive field center with increasing depolarization or hyperpolarization, according to cell type. If the image is small, i.e. not larger than the receptive field center, the horizontal cell response is dissipated through coupling and has little effect on the bipolar cell response. If the image is larger than the receptive field center, it will activate the opponent surround (through horizontal cells) to some extent no matter where it is placed. This will have the effect of reducing the apparent dimensions of the receptive field center, changing the form of the receptive field profile from a simple bell (monotonic) to a mexican hat (opponent surround). A corollary is that the response profile of a single bipolar cell to a moving black/white border, or of a linear array of bipolar cells crossing that edge perpendicularly, reflects edge-enhancement (Mach-band effect) (see e.g. Fain, 1980). Diffuse (or finely patterned but widespread) background illumination will speed up the kinetics of photoreceptor-bipolar synaptic transmission (Lam et al., 1978) and shift the operating curve (V-log I function) of the bipolar cell to higher intensities, thereby reducing its linear incremental sensitivity (Normann & Weblin, 1974, 1977). In sum, the achromatic horizontal-bipolar cell systems (rod or R-cone horizontals to a1 or b1 bipolars) permit maximal threshold sensitivity at the expense of spatial (and temporal) acuity in the dark (zero background), but enhance acuity at the expense of sensitivity in a well-lighted environment. They thus preserve or reinforce properties intrinsic to the photoreceptors that synapse upon those bipolar cells, but through neural transmission from distant photoreceptors that do not synapse upon them.

A major limitation of achromatic systems is that they fail to discriminate an object of one color against a background of a different color if they are equal in brightness. The major advantage of color vision, of course, is that such camouflage is made much more difficult; a bright orange goldfish, for example, is now readily detectable against bright green vegetation.

In a typical achromatic (or monochromatic) center-surround opponent system, as just described, light of any spectral distribution stimulates center and surround equally well, resulting in optimal response to focal illumination and enhancement of responses to edges. In a single color-opponent (e.g. R-on-center, G-off-surround) cell, however, the stimulus for one mechanism may be practically invisible to the other. Thus a red spot (against darkness) or a full red background may be equally effective. The uniqueness of such a cell is brought out by moving either a large red stimulus against a green background, or a red-green border; it is an exquisite detector of successive color contrast (including movement of a color border). It also should have best spatial (and temporal) acuity for red objects against green backgrounds, by analogy with achromatic center-surround opponent cells.

In double-color-opponent cells, including some carp bipolars described recently by Kaneko & Tachibana (1981) as well as some goldfish ganglion cells (Daw, 1968) and primate striate cortical cells (Michael, 1981), unlike achromatic or single color-opponent cells, achromatic stimuli of any size, shape, and location are poor stimuli. The response to chromatic stimuli is represented approximately by the sum of responses of complementary single-color-opponent cells to the same stimuli. Consider a R-on-G-off-center, R-off-G-on-surround cell. A red spot evokes an on-response, a red annulus an off-response and inhibition, and the two together cancel; complementary behaviors for green stimuli give the same nulling for diffuse illumination. These, then, are cells that are uniquely sensitive to color, size and configuration. They respond best to a small object of one color against a background of another color, especially if moving; they are good detectors of simultaneous color contrast, but not very good detectors of edges, even if chromatically contrasting. By comparison with single-opponent cells, double-opponent cells seem to be poor candidates for high spatial acuity; being rather insensitive to chromatically neutral stimuli and even chromatically contrasting edges, they appear to be best suited for detecting color per se. It may not be surprising, therefore, that double-color-opponent cells tend to have rather large receptive fields; the double-opponent ganglion cells described by Daw (1968) have the largest receptive field center, and the double-opponent bipolars described by Kaneko & Tachibana (1981) must be larger than the probably achromatic, small-field, type a1 and b1 mixed bipolars. Single - (and double-) color-opponent bipolars are likely to be driven, at least in part, by chromatically complex or C-type horizontal cells (Kaneko, 1973; Stell, 1979) and in part by chromatically opponent amacrine cells (Marc et al., 1978; Marc, 1980).

DEVELOPMENTAL PLASTICITY IN PHOTORECEPTOR-BIPOLAR CONNECTIVITY

In the teleostean as in the mammalian retina, the populations of most neurons are fixed in number and relative locations rather early in life. In teleosts, however, new cells of all types are added throughout life at the growing retinal margin; and even in the already mature central retina, rod photoreceptors are added steadily by mitotic division of in situ precursors (Johns, 1982; Kock, 1982). In goldfish, therefore, we may ask how the newly added rods are

added into pre-existing synaptic circuitry, and how retinal growth
and cell addition influence spatial acuity.

Rod-Bipolar Synapses in Mature Retinas. We have noted already
that rods contact horizontal cells of a single (all-rod) type and
bipolar cells of half a dozen (mixed rod-cone) types. The dendrites
enter the subsynaptic enclosure of the rod spherule through a narrow
aperture. Having been characterized by electron microscopical study
of silver chromate-impregnated (Stell et al., 1977) or HRP-injected
(Saito et al., 1983) cells, these dendrites can usually be classified by their form, dimensions, and mode of termination.

One could imagine a variety of synaptogenetic schemes by which
useful patterns of receptor-bipolar connections are established.
For example, each rod could contact a single dendritic branchlet
from each of the seven second-order neurons known to receive from
rods. This is clearly not the case. Stell and Lightfoot (1979)
counted dendrites entering rods in a random sample of 168 spherules
sectioned horizontally through the subsynaptic aperture (entryway).
We found as few as 4 and as many as 14 dendrites per rod, with a
mean of 7.65 and a 93% range (approximately $\pm$ 2 standard deviations)
of 5-10 dendrites per rod (figure 4). Since all the measurements
were made within a small area (1 mm^2), it is unlikely that the wide
variations reflect marked spatial inhomogeneities in bipolar cell
distribution. Furthermore, both Golgi and EM studies suggest that

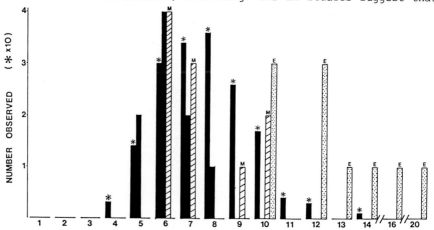

DENDRITES per ROD

Figure 4. Analyses of dendrites (rod horizontal and mixed rod-cone
bipolar cells) contacting goldfish rods. Dark bars: adult fish (11
cm. S.L.) from Ozark Fisheries; * = random sections through subsynaptic apertures of 168 spherules, unmarked = serial sections
through nine spherules. Light bars: fish provided by S.C. Sharma, M
= medium adult (9 cm. S.L.), E = stage 26 larva (60 hours post-
hatching), serial sections through ten spherules each. Note age-
dependent decreases in mean numbers of dendrites per rod.

branching of dendritic branchlets destined for rods, which might cause an apparent increase in number of second-order cells per rod, is rare.

We sought further insight into the rules of rod-bipolar synaptogenesis and synaptic regulation by analysis of rod synapses, serially ultrathin-sectioned and reconstructed and analyzed with computer assistance (Lightfoot et al, 1977; Stell and Lightfoot, 1979). We first reconstructed and analyzed nine rod spherules, with the enclosed dendrites and their receptor contacts, in "mature" goldfish (standard length ca. 11 cm.). These differed insignificantly from the larger, 168-rod survey population, having a mean total of 6.22 dendrites and a range of 5-8 dendrites per rod (figure 4). The mean numbers for specific classes of second-order neurons were 1.11 horizontal cells, 2.00 type a bipolars, and 3.11 type b bipolars. Although the variance was rather large, we were surprised to discover that in no instance did a rod fail to contact at least one each of these main classes of second-order cells. This analysis excluded, perhaps, the new hyperpolarizing bipolar of Saito and colleagues, our "a3" (see earlier), whose rod contacts were not known to us at the time; but the observed minimum of 4 dendrites per rod may indicate that dendrites of this bipolar cell type are treated separately and are always included as a fourth essential component.

Rod synaptogenesis appears to be rigidly programmed or regulated, therefore, to the extent that it provides each definitive or viable rod synapse with dendrites from at least one rod horizontal, one type a bipolar, one type b bipolar, and perhaps one type "a3" bipolar cell. Still the controls must be rather loose, since dendrites of bipolar cell subtypes a1, a2, b2 and b3 were often excluded, and supernumerary dendrites identifiable as rod horizontal, or b1 or b2 bipolar, were sometimes present.

What rules, beyond the minimum numerical requirement mentioned previously, might determine the amounts of specialized contact between rods and second-order cells? One might imagine, for example, that each rod makes available a fixed area of specialized contact of each type (i.e. for dendrites of each major class), so that the total area for each junctional type would be invariant with number of dendrites. At the other extreme each dendrite, independently or by interaction with the rod, might determine the area of junctional specialization, which in consequence would vary with the total number of dendrites of each type.

In our small sample, the area of rod-horizontal cell contact was highly variable and rather independent of number of horizontal cell dendrites. This could be explained by random, independent determinations of contact area by either rod or horizontal cell. The areas of rod-bipolar cell junctions per rod, however, showed a significant correlation with the numbers of dendrites, particularly in the case of the narrow-cleft junctions of type b bipolars. In this instance it may be that the rod sets a (randomly variable) total area of bipolar cell junctions and attracts or maintains a proportional number of dendrites, or that variable numbers of dendrites grow to the rod and add or induce proportional increments of junctional area.

Age-Dependent Patterns of Rod Synaptogenesis. A more direct approach to the problem of control of connectivity is to examine synaptogenesis in developing retina. Using serial electron micrography, we studied photoreceptor synaptogenesis in embryonic (pre-hatching) and larval (post-hatching) goldfish (Graf et al., 1979). At hatching, the only photoreceptors observed were well-differentiated cones. By 60 hours after hatching the first rod spherules could be detected. These early spherules were complex, containing synaptic ribbons and membrane specializations like those found in more mature retinas. Like adult rods, the larval rods contacted at least one each of the three major classes of second-order cells, with a significant preponderance of rod-bipolar over rod-horizontal cell contacts. Surprisingly, the number of dendrites invaginating each spherule was significantly greater in the 10 serially sectioned larval rods (range 10-20 per rod) than in the 9 serially sectioned adult rods (range 5-8 per rod) (figure 4). The difference in number was ascribable primarily to dendrites of type b bipolars, which were clearly more numerous in larval than in adult rods; statistically, the numbers of horizontal cell dendrites did not differ significantly, while the type a bipolar cell dendrites were probably more numerous in larval than adult rods.

This evidence confirms that in the early stages of embryonic-larval development, at least, rods are added to an initially all-cone receptor population. The large relative excess of larval over adult bipolar cell dendrites per rod suggests again that bipolar cells may play a more critical role than rods themselves in determining rod-bipolar cell connectivity. It also provides further evidence that synaptic connections of rods may change markedly during growth and maturation, although exactly how they change remains to be determined. On the one hand, the lack of overlap in connectivity patterns of larval and adult rods might suggest an age-dependent plasticity or remodeling, i.e., a progressive loss of bipolar cell dendrites from rod synapses with age. On the other hand, the larval rods are such a small fraction of the adult population that they might be missed in a random sampling of even hundreds of adult rods. The presence of an occasional adult synapse with far more than the usual number of dendrites (four with 11, three with 12, and one with 14 dendrites, fig. 4) is consistent with either interpretation; what is needed is a direct measurement of numbers of dendrites in newly formed rods at different ages.

Rod Addition in Adult Fish. Johns (1982) has documented clearly, by ^{3}H-thymidine labeling and autogradiographical localization of newly postmitotic cells, that rods are added to definitive, mature goldfish retina by mitosis of undifferentiated precursors in situ. She has suggested that rod precursors, but not definitive rods, are generated in the proliferative ring at the retinal margin. These precursors spend some time just proximal to the outer synaptic layer (i.e., among the horizontal cells), then migrate distally to the outer nuclear layer. There they may divide to form new rods or rod precursors.

We have confirmed Johns' observations in goldfish, including ^{3}H-thymidine-labeled animals kindly provided by Dr. S.C. Sharma, and in newborn live-bearing sea perch (Damalichthys vacca) obtained at the Friday Harbor (WA) Laboratories through the kindness of Mr. & Mrs. Bill Webb of Webb Camp Sea Farms. The results were particularly clear-cut in perch, which appear to undergo a growth spurt after birth and thus show large numbers of new, labeled rods throughout the retina at 2 days after ^{3}H-thymidine injection (figure 5). At the periphery there is a ring of heavily labeled undifferentiated cells. Just central from this ring a few labeled cells, presumably differentiating neurons of various types, are found in all layers except the outer nuclear layer. Central to this is a region containing no labeled cells at all. The remainder of the retina contains large numbers of newly differentiated rods, but no labeled neurons of any other kind.

Adult photoreceptor development at the retinal margins, therefore, recapitulates larval development in the retinal centre. First formed is a ring of differentiated cones plus undifferentiated rod precursors; subsequently these precursors differentiate into mature rods.

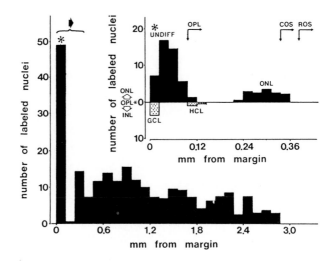

Figure 5. Rod genesis in mature retina of newborn sea perch, Damalichthys vacca, analyzed by ^{3}H-thymidine incorporation, survival for 48 hours at 16°C, fixation in aldehydes and OsO_4, and autoradiography of 1 µm epoxy sections. Main graph shows: large concentration of newly postmitotic neurons and precursors at retinal margin; adjacent ring containing few labeled cells; and disc of labeled cells (mostly rods) in central area including most of the retina. Inset shows expansion of far periphery, separating undifferentiated cells at margin (*UNDIFF) from cells in ganglion cell layer (GCL), horizontal cell layer (HCL; presumed rod precursors), and outer nuclear layer (ONL; differentiating rods). Farthest peripheral location of outer plexiform layer (OPL), cone outer segments (COS) and rod outer segments (ROS) is indicated by arrows.

Plasticity of Rod-Bipolar Cell Connectivity. We have investigated how newly formed rods are accommodated within the dendritic trees of pre-existing second-order neurons by analyzing the dendritic contacts of type bl bipolar cells (Kock et al., 1983). These cells were chosen because they are known to contact every rod within their dendritic field and because they are easily recognized and analyzed in Golgi preparations (Ishida et al., 1980). We made Golgi preparations of retinas from very small and very large fish, approximately 6 months and 5 years of age, respectively, embedded them in plastic, identified bl bipolars in 70 µm-thick vertical sections, and re-sectioned them serially at 0.5 µm in the plane of the photoreceptor terminals for light-microscopical analysis of their rod and cone contacts (Stell & Lightfoot, 1975; Stell & Lightfoot, 1980). The results are illustrated in figure 6.

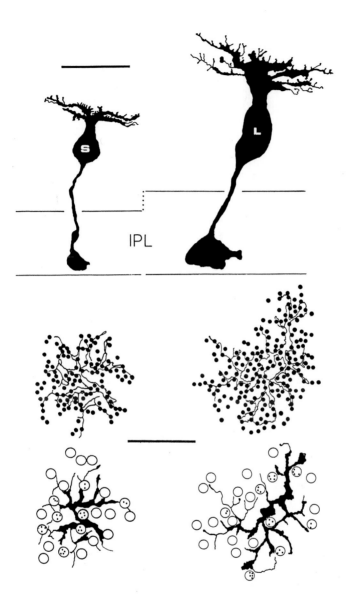

IPL

Figure 6. Rod and cone contacts of mixed rod-cone bipolar cell, type b1, in small (left, "S", ca. 6 mo.) and large (right, "L", ca. 5 yr.) goldfish, showing overall increase in cell dimensions, increases in number of rods contacted (dots), and constancy of cones contacted (open circles containing dots) with growth. Camera lucida drawings of Golgi preparations, in single thick vertical sections (above), and reconstruction of contacts in serial semithin sections (below). Bar = 20 µm.

During growth from 6 months to 5 years of age, the number of rod synapses onto each b1 bipolar increases by about 50%, from about 120 to 180 per cell. The added rods are accommodated into a bipolar cell dendritic tree that has grown by 54%, from about 1300 μm^2 in small retinas to 2000 μm^2 in large retinas. Irrespective of retinal size, therefore, the density of rod-b1 synapses remains constant at about one per 11 μm^2 (as does the density of the rods themselves, since the b1 bipolars appear to contact every rod). New rod synapses are added at the rate of approximately one per b1 bipolar per month.

The retina stretches with growth and so neurons of all types other than rods become more widely separated. The cone layer expands by approximately 19% during the growth period considered here; concomitantly the density of cones contacted by b1 bipolar cell dendrites decreases by 15%, from one per 158 μm^2 in small retinas to one per 187 μm^2 in large retinas. The numbers of cones contacted and not contacted, within the b1 bipolar cell's dendritic field, remain constant with growth. The cones contacted are the red-sensitive ones in either case.

It is obvious, then, that growth is accompanied by both cell addition and retinal expansion. Bipolar cell dendritic trees enlarge to keep pace with the increasing separation of the cones (and rods) that contact them. It seems likely that the b1 bipolars (and other second-order neurons) maintain contact with their original compliment of rods and cones. New rods are added, which, as we have now shown, make new synapses that are added to these old bipolars.

Observations on the properties of synaptic transmission from rods to bipolar cells (Ashmore & Falk, 1976, 1977; Lamb & Simon, 1977; Ashmore & Copenhagen, 1980) show that stochastic thermal isomerizations of rhodopsin generate a background of noise that accompanies light-evoked signals. Optimal signal detection requires discrimination of the light signal from thermal noise, and the signal: noise ratio might be improved by increasing the number of synaptic channels. Whether or not this is the case is in doubt. The only hard data on this subject (Power & Bassi, 1981, 1982), "suggest that goldfish retinal ganglion cells maintain a constant signal-to-noise criterion during growth", and one might suppose that this reflects the properties of rod-bipolar cell assemblies from which the ganglion cells recieve. It might therefore be true, paradoxically, that the addition of rods is itself somehow responsible for keeping absolute sensitivity contant as the eye grows.

Powers and Easter (1978) determined the absolute sensitivity of 12–14 cm goldfish to be one quantum incident per 2000–4000 rods ($\lambda =$ 532 nm) or 220 R cones ($\lambda =$ 636 nm). The dendritic tree of a b1 bipolar cell, which receives from about 200 rods and 8 R cones, covers an area on the order of $1.0 - 1.5 \times 10^{-3}$ mm^2 (data from Ishida et al., 1980). If the coverage factor of b1 bipolars is unity, and if double-color-opponent ganglion cells integrate from them over an area of about 2 mm^2 (r^2 0.8 mm; Daw, 1968), then there are about 1300 – 2000 b1 bipolars per ganglion cell center. At either rod or R cone threshold, therefore, one quantum is incident per 15–25 b1 bipolar cells, and about 50–100 quanta are incident per double-color-opponent ganglion cell center. Since only a small fraction of b1 bipolars receive from quantum-activated rods or cones at threshold, the double-opponent ganglion cells are more likely than b1 bipolar cells to be the integrating units responsible for threshold. The probable invariance of b1–ganglion cell connectivity with growth might then account for the invariance of threshold with growth.

Another functional consequence of the observed patterns of retinal growth returns us to the subject of spatial acuity. Since the teleostean retina grows not only by stretching but also by peripheral cell addition, the visual angle subtended by the distance between two cones (or the dendritic tree of a single second-order cell) decreases with growth. This should result in a steady increase of visual acuity with growth. While this hypothesis has not been examined in goldfish, it is supported by data in other teleosts (Yamanouchi, 1956; Baerends et al., 1960) and is undoubtedly true in goldfish as well.

RETINAL STRUCTURE AND SPATIAL ACUITY

Structural Constraints. One would expect intuitively some correlation between the structure and structural interconnections of retinal cells, on the one hand, and the functional properties of those cells in spatial vision on the other. For example, there is an obvious progression from numerous, densely packed photoreceptors to sparse, widely scattered ganglion cells, matched by a progression from small to large functional receptive fields (figure 7). As summarized early in this paper, goldfish cones are separated by distances of 10–25 µm, and their functional receptive fields are probably on the order of 100 µm in diameter; the smallest goldfish bipolars are probably distributed at center-center distances of

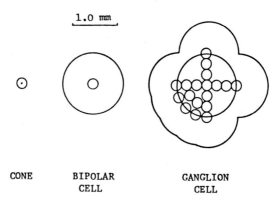

Figure 7. Schematic representation of receptive field dimensions at three stages of spatial information processing in goldfish retina. Left, cone separation (spot) and probable summation area or spread function (circle). Center, bipolar cell receptive field center and surround. Right, double-color-opponent ganglion cell centers for red (inner circle containing small circles, representing summation of bipolar cell centers) and green (outer perimeter representing summation of bipolar cell surrounds). 1 mm on retina equals approximately 15 degrees visual angle. Redrawn and modified from Raynauld (1975).

about 35 μm with little or no dendritic overlap, and their receptive field centers (estimated from those of closely related but larger carp) must measure on the order of 100-200 μm; ganglion cells are much larger, having dendritic tree diameters of 100-350 μm and more in the closely related crucian carp, and receptive field centers on the order of 200-2200 μm in most cases.

Spatial Correlations. Which of these dimensions is best related to spatial acuity? The answer varies according to how acuity is measured.

The finest dimensions are indicated by grating methods, which suggest that acuity (grating half-period) may be of similar dimensions whether determined by visual behavior, ganglion cell physiology, or intercone distances (Table 2).

Somewhat larger dimensions are indicated by point-spread functions determined for visual behavior or photoreceptor physiology, which are correlated with the dimensions (1) of dendritic trees of the smaller bipolar and ganglion cells and (2) of receptive field centers for cones and bipolar cells determined by static methods (Table 3). It is evident, however, that as one ascends toward the brain, increasing nonlinearities can make the receptive

TABLE 2

BEST GRATING ACUITY (half-period)

Indicator	Reference	"Acuity" Deg. vis. angle	μm on retina
Behavior	Northmore & Dvorak '79	0.2 – 0.4	13.6 – 25.8
GC Physiology (grating)	Schwassmann '75	0.3	20
Cone-cone separation	Stell & Harosi '76	0.2 – 0.4	10 – 25
Cone telodendron	Lockhart & Stell '79	0.4	25

fields substantially narrower for spatially complex than for spatially simple stimuli (figure 8). Such measurements also reinforce
the notion that hyperpolarizing bipolars, being more cone-dominated,
are part of a higher-acuity system (Table 4).

Still larger dimensions are suggested by methods that rely upon
spatial summation areas (Ricco's Law). Under both scotopic and
photopic conditions, Ricco's areas determined behaviorally are
closely correlated with those determined for the smallest receptive
field centers of ganglion cells; the dynamic receptive fields of
bipolar cells and the dendritic spreads of the smallest ganglion
cells are also of the same order (Table 5).

There are, finally, some measures of spatial acuity for which
no good correlations are apparent between behavioral, physiological,
and anatomical dimensions. These are summarized in Table 6.

Retinal Basis of Acuity. Obviously "spatial acuity" compre-
hends a number of different phenomena which have different func-

TABLE 3

POINT SPREAD FUNCTION (DERIVED)

Indicator	Reference	"Acuity" Deg. vis. angle	μm on retina
Behavior (grating) (1/2 max-max)	Northmore & Dvorak '79	0.6 – 1.6	40 – 100
SGC anatomy	Kock & Reuter '78	1.6	100
BC anatomy	Ishida et al, '80	0.6 – 1.6	40 – 100
	Saito & Kujiraoka '82	0.8 – 1.5	56 – 90
	Saito et al. '83	0.9 – 1.7	65 – 114
	Naka & Carraway '75 (Catfish)		75 – 150
BC physiology (dynamic)	Powers & Arnett '81 (Catfish)		94 – 300
BC physiology (static)	Kaneko '73	≥1.6	100 – 200
Cone physiology (static)	Burkhart '77 (Perch)		100
	(Baylor & Hodgkin '73 (Turtle)		50 – 150
	Lasater '82a (Catfish) (grating: 1/2 max-max)		70 – 130

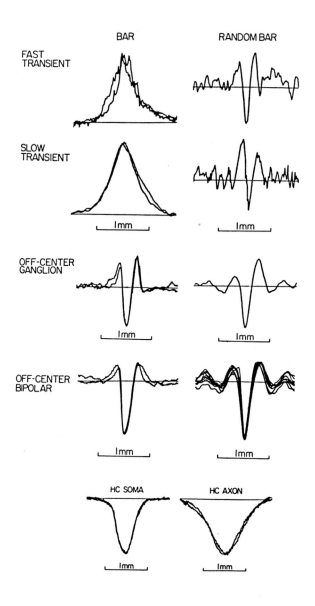

Figure 8. Reconstructions of receptive field profiles by spatial white-noise (single bar and pseudo-random bar grating) analysis. Note absence of spatial sharpening in responses of horizontal cell (HC) and in slow- and fast- transient responses to single bars. Note presence of sharpening, which preserves narrowest cone receptive field dimensions, in responses of OFF-bipolar and ganglion cell, and in responses of transient cells to complex (random bar) stimulus. Adapted from Davis and Naka (1980).

TABLE 4

ACUITIES OF ON vs. OFF SYSTEMS
(Powers & Arnett, '81)

Type of Cell	ON (depol.)	OFF (hyperpol.)
Bipolar	108±21	94±16
Ganglion	395±91	312±22

tional bases in retinal circuitry. Grating acuity for behavior and
ganglion cell function is larger than optical limits of resolution
but approaches intercone distances. Point-spread functions
(including spatiotemporal white-noise function) suggest that the
receptive fields of cones for complex, moving stimuli are strongly
influenced by interactions such as electrical coupling and are
therefore substantially larger than intercone distances. The
smallest second- and third-order units seem to preserve the dimensions of cone point-spread functions, probably in part by means of
antagonistic center-surround interactions. It is likely that the
small-cell pathways have been largely overlooked (through sampling
bias) in microelectrode studies of goldfish ganglion cells. Ricco's
areas appear to be determined by the spatially summing properties of
ganglion cell dendritic trees, the behavioral limit being due to the
largest, rod-dominated ganglion cells scotopically and the smallest,
cone-dominated ganglion cells photopically. The spatially summing
properties of photoreceptors and bipolars seem not to contribute
directly to Ricco's areas. Chromatic effects on acuity, which seem
likely from a consideration of color-opponent organization in bipolar and ganglion cells, have as yet to be investigated functionally
or physiologically. This should be a fascinating and fruitful
avenue for further study.

TABLE 5

RICCO'S AREA

Indicator	Reference	"Acuity" Deg. vis. angle	"Acuity" μm on retina
Behavior (Photopic)	Northmore '77	≥3-5	200-350
GC physiology (smallest fields)	Beauchamp & Lovasik '73	3-5	180-350
	Schellart & Spekreijse '76		
	Davis & Naka '80		
	Lasater '82b		
	Powers & Arnett '81		170-400
LGC	Kock & Reuter '78	≤5	≤350
BC physiology (dynamic)	Davis & Naka '80 (Catfish)		185-190
HC Physiology (dynamic)	Powers & Arnett '81 (Catfish)		300
	Davis & Naka '80 (Catfish)		500-800
*Behavior (scotopic)	Northmore '77	30°	ca. 2200
*GC physiology	Daw '68	ca. 30°	≤2200

TABLE 6

MISCELLANEOUS

| Indicator | Reference | "Acuity" | |
		Deg. vis. angle	µm on retina
*GC Physiology	Daw '68	21.6–25.6	1350–1600
(Double-opponent)			
GC Anatomy	Naka & Carraway '75		ca. 500–1000
	(catfish)		
BC Physiology	Saito & Kujiraoka '82	ca. 7–8	500
(Static)	Saito et al. '83	ca. 9–10	700

*Non-corresponding for cones but good fit for rods (Northmore '77)

ACKNOWLEDGEMENTS

The authors gratefully acknowledge the technical assistance of Mrs. Artee Karkhanis and the secretarial work of Mrs. Mary Pollack. These studies were supported by grants from the U.S. Public Health Service, The Medical Research Council (Canada), and The Alberta Heritage Foundation for Medical Research.

REFERENCES

Ashmore, J.F. and D.R. Copenhagen. 1980. Different postsynaptic events in two types of retinal bipolar cell. Nature. Lond.) 288; 84–86.

Ashmore, J.F. and G. Falk. 1976. Absolute sensitivity of rod bipolar cells in a dark-adapted retina. Nature (Lond.) 263; 248–249.

Ashmore, J.F. and G. Falk. 1977. Dark noise in retinal bipolar cells and stability of rhodopsin in rods. Nature (Lond.) 270; 69–71.

Baerends, G.P., B.E. Bennema and A.A. Vogelzang. 1960. Über die Änderung der Sehschärfe mit dem Wachstum bei Aequidens portalegrenis (Hensel) (Pisces, Cichlidae). Zool. Jahrb. Abt. Sept. Okt. 88; 67–78.

Baylor, D.A., M.G.F. Fuortes and P.M. O'Bryan. 1971. Receptive fields of cones in the retina of the turtle. J. Physiol. (Lond.) 214; 265–294.

Baylor, D.A. & R. Fettiplace. 1977. Transmission from photoreceptors to ganglion cells in the retina of the turtle. In: Vertebrate Photoreception (B.B. Barlow and P. Fatt, eds.). Academic Press, London & New York. pp. 193–203.

Baylor, D.A. and A.L. Hodgkin. 1973. Detection and resolution of visual stimuli by turtle photoreceptors. J. Physiol. 234; 163–198.

Beauchamp, R.D. and N.W. Daw. 1972. Rod and cone input to single goldfish optic nerve fibers. Vision Res. 12; 1201–1212.

Beauchamp, R.D. and J.V. Lovasik. 1973. Blue mechanism response of single goldfish optic fibers. J. Neurophysiol. 36; 925–939.

Burkhardt, D.A. 1977. Responses and receptive-field organization of cones in perch retinas. J. Neurophysiol. 40; 53–62.

Cajal, S.R.Y. 1892. La retine des vertebres. Cellule 91 121–225.

Cohen, A.I. 1972. Rods and cones. In: Physiology of Photoreceptor Organs. (Handb. Sens. Physiol. VII/2). (M.G.F. Fuortes, ed.) Springer-Verlag, Berlin. pp. 63–110.

Copenhagen, D.R. and W.G. Owen. 1980. Current-voltage relations in the rod photoreceptor network of the turtle retina. J. Physiol. (Lond.) 308; 159-184.

Davis, G.W. and K.-I. Naka. 1980. Spatial organizations of catfish retinal neurons. I. Single- and random-bar stimulation. J. Neurophysiol. 43; 807-831.

Daw, N.W. 1968. Color-coded ganglion cells in the goldfish retina: extension of their receptive fields by means of new stimuli. J. Physiol. 223; 449-460. Drujan, D.B. and M. Laufer. 1982. The S-Potential. Alan R. Liss, New York. 319.

Easter, S.S. Jr., P.R. Johns, and L.R. Baumann, 1977. Growth of the adult goldfish eye. I. Optics. Vision Res. 17; 469-477.

Famiglietti, E.V. Jr., A Kaneko and M. Tachibana. 1977. Neuronal architecture of on and off pathways to ganglion cells in carp retina. Science 198; 1267-1269.

Famiglietti, E.V. Jr., and H. Kolb. 1976. Structural basis for "on"-and "off"-center responses in retinal ganglion cells. Science. 194; 193-195.

Fain, G.L. 1980. Integration by spikeless neurons in the retina. In: Neurones Without Impulses: Their Significance in Vertebrate and Invertebrate Nervous Systems. (BMH Bush and A. Roberts, eds.). Cambridge University Press, London, pp. 29-59.

Gold, G.H. 1981. Photoreceptor coupling: Its mechanism and consequences. In: Molecular Mechanisms of Photoreceptor Transduction (Current Topics in Membranes and Transport, vol. 15) (W.H. Miller, ed.). Academic Press, New York, pp. 59-89. Graf, S.A., W.K. Stell and S.C. Sharma. 1979. Invest. Ophthal. Vis. Sci. (Suppl.). 19; 82.

Ishida, A.T., W.K. Stell and D.O. Lightfoot. 1980. J. Comp. Neurol. 191; 315-335.

Johns, P.R. 1982. Formation of photoreceptors in larval and adult goldfish. J. Neurosci. 2; 178-198.

Kaneko, A. 1973. Receptive field organization of bipolar and amacrine cells in the goldfish retina. J. Physiol. 235; 133-153.

Kaneko, A. and M. Tachibana. 1981. Retinal bipolar cells with double colour-opponent receptive fields. Nature (Lond.) 293; 220-222.

Kock, J.-H. 1982. Neuronal addition and retinal expension during growth of the crucian carp eye. J. Comp Neurol. 219; 264-274.

Kock, J.-H., A. Karkhanis and W.K. Stell. 1983. The bl bipolar cell: Evidence for synaptic plasticity in goldfish retina. Invest Ophthal. Vis. Sci. (Suppl.) 23; in press.

Kock, J.-H. and T. Reuter. 1978. Retinal ganglion cells in the crucian carp (Carassius carassius). II. Overlap, shape and tangential orientation of dendritic trees. J. comp. Neurol. 179; 549-568.

Kolb, H. 1970. Organization of the outer plexiform layer of the primate retina: Electron microscopy of Golgi-impregnated cells. Proc. Roy. Soc. Lond. B.258; 261-283.

Lam, D.M.K., E.M. Lasater and K-I. Naka. 1978. Gamma-aminobutyric acid: a neurotransmitter candidate for some horizontal cells of the catfish retina. Proc. Nat. Acad. Sci. USA. 75; 6310-6313.

Lamb, T.D., and E.J. Simon. 1977. Analysis of electrical noise in turtle cones. J. Physiol. (Lond.) 272; 435-468.

Lasansky, A. 1971. Synaptic organization of cone cells in the turtle retina. Phil. Trans. Roy. Soc. Lond. B262; 365-381.

Lasater, E.M. 1982a. A white-noise analysis of responses and receptive fields of catfish cones. J. Neurophysiol. 47; 1057-1068.

Lasater, E.M. 1982b. Spatial receptive fields of catfish retinal ganglion cells. J. Neurophysiol. 48; 823-835.

Levick, W.R. and L.N. Thibos. 1982. Analysis of orientation bias in cat retina. J. Physiol. (Lond.) 329; 243-261.

Lightfoot, D.O., W.K. Stell, M.J. Shantz and G.D. McCann. 1977. Computer-aided reconstruction of rod-synapses in goldfish retina. Soc. Neurosci. Abstract. 3; 390.

Lockhart, M. and W.K. Stell. 1979. Invaginating telodendria: a pathway for color-specific interconnections between goldfish cones. Invest. Ophthal. Vis. Sci. (Suppl.) 19; 82.

Marc, R.E. 1980. Retinal colour channels and their neurotransmitters. In: Colour Deficiencies V. (G. Verriest, ed.) Adam Hilger, London, pp. 15-29.

Marc, R.E. 1982. Spatial organization of neurochemically classified interneurons of the goldfish retina. I. Local patterns. Vision Res. 22; 589-608.

Marc, R.E. and H.G. Sperling. 1976. Chromatic organization of the goldfish cone mosaic. Vision Res. 16; 1211-1224.

Marc, R.E. and H.G. Sperling. 1977. The Chromatic organization of primate cones. Science. 196; 454-456.

Marc, R.E., W.K. Stell, D. Bok and D.M.K. Lam. 1978. GABA-ergic pathways in the goldfish retina. J. Comp. Neurol. 182; 221-245.

Michael, C.R. 1978. Color vision mechanisms in monkey striate cortex: dual-opponent cells with concentric receptive fields. J. Neurophysiol. 41; 572-588.

Nagy, A., W.K. Stell and D.O. Lightfoot. 1983. A freeze-fracture study of photoreceptor synapses in goldfish retina. Submitted for publication.

Naka, K.-I. and N.R.G. Carraway. 1975. Morphological and functional identification of catfish retinal neurons. I. Classical morphology. J. Neurophysiol. 38; 53-71.

Normann, R.A. and F.S. Werblin. 1974. Control of retinal sensitivity. I. Light and dark adaptation of vertebrate rods and cones. J. Gen. Physiol. 63; 37-61.

Northmore, D.P.M. 1977. Spatial summation and light adaptation in the goldfish visual system. Nature (Lond.) 268; 450-451.

Northmore, D.P.M. and C.A. Dvorak. Contrast sensitivity and acuity of the goldfish. Vision Re. 19; 255-261.

Parthe, V. 1982. Horizontal cells in the teleost retina. In: The S-Potential. (B.D. Drujan and M. Laufer, eds.). Alan R. Liss, New York. pp. 31-49.

Powers, M.K. and C.J. Bassis. 1981. Absolute visual threshold is determined by the proportion of stimulated rods in the growing goldfish retina. Sco. Neurosci. Abstracts 7; 541.

Powers, M.K. and C.J. Bassi. 1982. Rod threshold in the growing goldfish. This Symposium.

Powers, M.K. and S.S. Easter, Jr. 1982. The Eye. In: Fish. Neurobiology and Behavior (R.E. Davis and R.G. Northcutt, eds.) U. Mich. Press, Ann Arbor. In press.

Powers, R.L. and D.W. Arnett. 1981. Spatio-temporal cross-correlation analysis of catfish retinal neurons. Biol. Cybernet. 41; 179-196.

Raynauld, J.-P. 1972. Goldfish retina: Sign of the rod input in opponent color ganglion cells. Science. 177; 85-86.

Raynauld, J.-P. 1975. A model for the ganglionic receptive field organization. In: Vision in Fishes. New Approaches in Research. (M.A. Ali, ed.) Plenum, New York. pp. 91-98.

Saito, T., H. Kondo and J. Toyoda. 1979. Ionic mechanisms of two types of on-center bipolar cells in the carp retina. 1. The responses to central illumination. J. Gen. Physiol. 73; 73-90.

Saito, T and T. Kujinraoka. 1982. Physiological and morphological identification of two types of on-center bipolar cell in the carp retina. J. Comp Neurol. 205; 161-170.

Saito, T., T. Kujiraoka and T. Yonaha. 1983. Connections between photoreceptors and horseradish perioxidase-injected bipolar cells in the carp retina. 4th Taniguchi Symposium, in press.

Schellart, N.A.M. and H. Spekreijse. 1972. Dynamic characteristics of retinal ganglion cell responses in goldfish. J. Gen. Physiol. 59; 1-21.

Scholes, J.H. 1975. Colour receptors, and their synaptic connections, in the retinal of a cyprinid fish. Phil. Trans. Roy. Soc. B.270; 61-118.

Scholes, J.H. 1976. Neuronal connections and cellular arrangement in the fish retina. In: Neural Principles in Vision (F. Zettler and Re. Weiler, eds.) Springer-Verlag, Berlin. pp. 63-93.

Schwassmann, H.O. 1975. Refractive state, accommodation, and resolving power of the fish eye. In: Vision in Fishes (M.Aa. Ali, Ed.). Plenum, New York. pp. 279-288.

Shantz, M.J. 1978. Computational morphology: Three-dimensional computer graphics for electron microscopy. IEEE Trans. Biomed. Eng. 25; 99-103.

Stell, W.K. 1967. The structure and relationships of horizontal cells and photoreceptor-bipolar synaptic complexes in goldfish retina. Amer. J. Anat. 121; 401-423.

Stell, W.K. 1976. Functional polarization of horizontal cell dendrites in goldfish retina. Invest. Ophthal. 15; 895-908.

Stell, W.K. 1979. Inputs to bipolar cell dendrites in goldfish retina. Sens. Proc. 2; 339-349.

Stell, W.K. 1980. Photoreceptor-specific synaptic pathways in goldfish retina: a world of colour, a wealth of connections. In: Colour Vision Deficiencies V. (G. Verriest, ed.). Hilger, London, pp. 1-12.

Stell, W.K. and F.I. Harosi. 1976. Cone structure and visual pigment content in the retina of the goldfish. Vision Res. 16; 647-657.

Stell, W.K., A.T. Ishida and D.L. Lightfoot. 1977. Structural basis for ON- and OFF-center responses in retinal bipolar cells. Science 198; 1269-1271.

Stell, W.K., R. Kretz and D.O. Lightfoot. 1982. Horizontal cell connectivity in goldfish. In: The S-Potential. (B.D. Drujan and M. Laufer, eds.). Alan R. Liss, New York. pp. 51-75.

Stell, W.K. and D.O. Lightfoot. 1975. Color-specific interconnections of cones and horizontal cells in the retina of the goldfish. J. Comp. Neurol. 159; 473-502.

Stell, W.K. and D.O. Lightfoot. 1979. Computer-aided reconstruction and analysis of goldfish rod synapses. Seitai-no-Kagaku 30; 173-177, (Japanese transl. A. Kaneko).

Svaetichin, G. 1953. The cone action potential. Acta. Physiol. Scand. 29. (Suppl.) 106; 465-600.

Van Hawsendonck, E. and L. Missotten. 1979. Synaptic contacts of the horizontal cells in the retina of the marine teleost, Callionymus lyra L. J. Comp. Neurol. 184; 167-191.

Wagner, H.-J. 1978. Cell types and connectivity patterns in mosaic retinas. Advan. Anat. Embryol. Cell Biol 55(3); 1-81.

Wagner, H.-J. and P.T. Speck. 1982. Computer reconstruction of HRP-injected horizontal cells reveals new connectivity patterns in fish retina. Naturwiss. 69; 143-144.

Werblin, F.S. 1974. Control of retinal sensitivity. II. Lateral interactions at the outer plexiform layer. J. Gen. Phyiol. 63; 62-87.

Werblin, F.S. 1977. Synaptic interactions mediating bipolar response in the retina of the tiger salamander. In: Vertebrate Photoreception (H.B. Barlow and P. Fatt, eds.). Academic Press, London and New York. pp. 205-230.

Localization of Neuropeptides in the Adult and Developing Retina

N.C. Brecha and H.J. Karten

The presence of neuropeptide activity in the retina was first reported over 25 years ago by Duner et al (1954) who described the presence of substance P biological activity in mammalian retinal extracts. However, not until recently, has there been a detailed documentation of the presence and localization of peptide systems within the vertebrate retina (see Brecha, 1983; Karten and Brecha, 1982; Brecha and Karten, 1983 for reviews). This renewed interest is no doubt a direct result of general interest in nervous system and gut peptides as well as the attractiveness of the retina for detailed anatomical, physiological and biochemical studies.

The vertebrate retina has proven to be amendable to detailed experimental study for several reasons. First, the morphology of the retina is well understood and it is characterized by a clear and distinct laminar organization. Morphological studies have demonstrated that the retina contains a limited number of major cell types which can be characterized by both the location of their soma as well as the pattern of arborization of their processes (Cajal, 1893). In addition, ultrastructural studies have demonstrated the synaptic relationships of these neuronal cell types to one another. Second, electrophysiological studies have characterized the responses of the retina as a whole and its major cell types to light stimulation. Finally, the retina is readily accessible to experimental manipulation and can easily be used in situ, in vivo and in vitro for a variety of physiological, pharmacological and biochemical studies. It is the combination of all these factors which provides the opportunity to better assess the functional role of presumed transmitter substances in visual processes and, more generally, to better understand what functional role or roles these substances play in neuronal processes within the nervous system.

In this chapter evidence for the presence, localization and

possible functions of neuropeptides in the adult and developing retina will be reviewed.

PRESENCE OF NEUROPEPTIDES IN THE VERTEBRATE RETINA

Bioassay, immunoassay and immunohistochemical studies have firmly established the presence of peptide-like substances in the retinas of all vertebrate species studied to date (Table 1). Using these techniques good evidence for at least 12 peptides have been described. Undoubtedly, several more peptide-like substances will be reported in the retina in the near future since there is currently a great interest in the identification of new biologically active peptides in both the gut and nervous system. The best evidence to date suggests that several neuropeptides are present in the retina of any one species. However, not all of the peptides that have been found to be present in the retina of one vertebrate species will necessarily be found in the retina of another vertebrate species (Table 2). Moreover, as detailed below, both the retinal content of the peptide-like substances and the morphological appearance of the peptide-containing cells differ for each vertebrate species. Since the amino acid composition and sequence of the immunoreactive peptide-like substances found in the retina are unknown, except for somatostatin in the bovine retina (Marshak et al, 1982), it is appropriate to refer to these substances using such modifiers as "like" or "immunoreactive."

1) Bioassay Studies

Bioassay studies first described substance P-like (SP) bio-activity in dog and bovine retinal extracts (Duner et al, 1954). This study, using a smooth muscle (ileum) bioassay preparation, demonstrated high SP bioactivity in these retinas. A subsequent study, using a similar preparation, reported low SP bioactivity in bovine retinal extracts and that the majority of SP bioactivity was present in optic nerve extracts (Winder and Patsalos, 1974). Using a somatostatin bioassay system, recent studies have demonstrated that crude retinal extracts or immunoaffinity-purified retinal immu-noreactive somatostatin-like (SRIF) extracts from either rat or human retina will inhibit in a dose-related manner the release of growth hormone from anterior pituitary cell cultures (Rorstad et al, 1979, 1980). The inhibition of growth hormone release by retinal extracts is similar to that produced by synthetic somatostatin-14, supporting the suggestion that somatostatin is present in these retinas. To date, no other neuropeptides such as enkephalin, cholecystokinin or vasactive intestinal polypeptide which are present in the retina, as evidence by immunoassay or immunohistochemical studies, have been tested in a biological assay system. These biological assay systems are important because they provide an independent corroboration of the presence of the peptide-like substance in the retina.

2) Immunoassay Studies

Using radioimmunoassay techniques, the presence of at least ten neuropeptides have been described in the retinas of various vertebrate species (Tables 1 and 2). Cholecystokinin-like (CCK), enkephalin-like (ENK), SP, SRIF, thyrotropin releasing hormone-like (TRH) immunoreactivity are reported to be present in the retinas of representative vertebrate species (Brecha, 1983; Brecha et al, 1981A, 1982A; Buckerfield et al, 1981; Eiden et al, 1980; Martino et al, 1980; Kanazawa and Jessell, 1976; Reubi and Jessell, 1978; Osborne et al, 1981; Rorstad et al, 1979, 1980; Schaeffer et al, 1977; Unger et al, 1981; Yamada et al, 1980, 1981). ENK immunoreactivity has for the most part, only been detected in non-mammalian retinal extracts by radioimmunoassay (Jackson et al, 1980; Humbert et al, 1979), although recently, the presence of ENK immunoreactivity in the guinea pig retina by immunohistochemistry and radioimmunoassay has been reported (Altschuter et al, 1982; Mosinger et al, 1982). In addition, β-endorphin-like (β-END), glucagon-like (GLU), luteinizing releasing hormone-like (LRH), neurotensin-like (NT) and vasoactive intestinal polypeptide-like (VIP) immunoreactivity has been described in the retina of just one or two different vertebrate species (Brecha, 1983; Brecha et al, 1981A, 1982A; Jackson et al, 1980; Unger et al, 1981).

The retinal content of immunoreactive peptides including CCK, SP and SRIF range from very low to moderate in comparison to such peptide rich regions of the central nervous system as the hypothala-

TABLE 1

NEUROPEPTIDE-LIKE ACTIVITY OR IMMUNOREACTIVITY IN THE VERTEBRATE RETINA

	Bioassay	Radioimmunoassay	Chromatography	Immunohistochemistry
APP				x
CCK		x	x	x
ENK		x	x	x
β-END		x		x
FMRF-NH$_2$				x
GLU		x	x	x
LRF		x		x
NT		x		x
SP	x	x	x	x
SRIF	x	x	x	x
TRH		x	x	
VIP		x	x	x

TABLE 2

PRESENCE OF NEUROPEPTIDE-LIKE IMMUNOREACTIVITY IN THE RETINA OF VARIOUS VERTEBRATES BASED ON RADIOIMMUNOASSAY AND/OR IMMUNOHISTOCHEMICAL EVIDENCE*

	SP	ENK	SRIF	NT	VIP	GLU	CCK
-FISH-							
Goldfish (Carassius auratus)	+	+	+	+		+	+
Pile Perch (Damanichthys vacca)	+	+	+				
Cohoe salmon	+	+					
Sturgeon poacher	+						
Plainfin midshipman (Porichthys pacifica)	+						
Surfsmelt (Hypomesus pretisus)	+						
Rockfish (Sevastes caurinus)	+	+					
Channel catfish		+					
Carp	+	+	+			+	
-AMPHIBIANS-							
Xenopus laevis	+						
Toad (Bufo marinus)	+		+				
Frog (Rana pipiens)	+	+	+	+	+		
Bullfrog (Rana catesbeiana)							
Tiger Salamander (Ambysoma tigrinum)	+	+					
Mudpuppy (Necturus maculosus)	+	+	+	+	+	+	+
-REPTILES-							
Turtle (Chrysemys scripta)	+	+		+		+	
Lizard (Anolis carolinensis)	+	+					
Lizard (Uta stansburiana)	+						
Lizard (Gecko gecko)	+	+					
-BIRDS-							
Pigeon (Columba livia)	+	+	+	+	+	+	
Chicken (Gallus domesticus)	+	+	+	+	+	+	
-MAMMALS-							
Rat	+		+		+	+	
Rabbit	+		+		+		
Cat	+		+		+		
Guinea Pig	+						
New World monkey (Saimmira sciureus)	+		+		+		
Old World monkey (Macaca nemestrima)	+		+		+		
(Macaca facicularis)	+		+		+		
Human	+		+				

*A blank in this table does not necessarily indicate the particular neuropeptide is absent from the retina.

mus, basal ganglia and brainstem (Eskay et al, 1980; Kanazawa and Jessell, 1976; Reubi and Jessell, 1978; Rorstad et al, 1979; Yamada et al, 1980, 1981). For example SRIF content in the retina is less than SRIF content in the optic tectum, hypothalamus and brainstem (Brownstein et al, 1975; Kobayashi et al, 1977; Rorstad et al, 1979, 1980; Unger et al, 1981; Yamada et al, 1980) and comparable to that in the rat pineal, cerebellum and substantia nigra (Brownstein et al, 1975; Kobayashi et al, 1977). It is noteworthy that a marked variance in the retinal content of immunoreactive peptides has also been observed among vertebrate species. The wide variance in the reported retinal immunoreactive peptide content appears to be genuine in that several groups have independently obtained similar findings. For instance, retinal SRIF content differs between gold-fish, frog, rat and rabbit retinas (Eskay et al, 1980; Rorstad et al, 1979; Unger et al, 1981; Yamada et al, 1980). Some of this variability may be due to technical differences such as tissue preparation and extraction, although the exact biological reasons for these differences is not as yet known.

Gel filtration and/or high pressure liquid chromatographic techniques have been used to further characterize the nature of retinal peptide-like substances. To date, the techniques have pro-vided evidence for the presence of CCK, ENK, GLU, SP and SRIF pep-tides in the vertebrate retina (Brecha et al, 1982A; Eskay et al, 1981; Humbert et al, 1979; Osborne et al, 1981; Rorstad et al, 1979; Yamada et al, 1980, 1981). These techniques have also been used to determine the amino acid composition and sequence of SRIF in the bovine retina (Marshak et al, 1982). Examples of this type of analysis which provide for a better understanding of the nature of the peptide-like substances present in the retina are given below.

Immunoreactive SRIF extracted from goldfish and rat retinas co-eluted with synthetic somatostatin-14 on Sephadex G25 or G50 (Rorstad et al, 1979; Shapiro et al, 1979; Yamada et al, 1980) suggesting the presence of somatostatin-14 in these retinas. In addition, a second SRIF immunoreactive peak, which is larger than somatostatin-14 and likely corresponding to somatostatin-28 has been reported in retinal extracts of goldfish, frogs, chickens and cows (Yamada et al, 1980; Marshak et al, 1982). The amino acid composi-tion and sequence of the larger retinal SRIF has recently been determined in bovine retina (Marshak et al, 1982). Retinal SRIF-immunoreactive extracts, isolated by a somatostatin affinity column, subsequently purified by high pressure liquid chromatography and analyzed by Edman degradation for its amino acid sequence was found to share the same amino acid composition and sequence as hypothala-mic somatostatin-28 (Esch et al, 1980; Schally et al, 1980). These studies thus demonstrate the presence of at least two molecular forms of somatostatin in the vertebrate retina.

In conclusion, both radioimmunoassay and chromatography studies have provided good evidence for the presence of several different neuropeptides within the retina. Radioimmunmnoassay studies have suggested these retinal immunoreactive substances are similar if not identical to known biologically active gut and nervous system peptides. Chromatography studies generally support this conclusion. In addition to the documentation of the presence of neuropeptides in the vertebrate retina, a great deal of information on the morphological localization of these substances has been obtained using immunohistochemical techniques.

3) Immunohistochemical Studies

Immunohistochemical studies have described the localization of nine neuropeptides including ENK, SP, SRIF and VIP in both mammalian and non-mammalian retinas (Tables 1 and 2) (Brecha, 1983; Brecha et al, 1979, 1980, 1981A, 1982A, 1982B; Buckerfield et al, 1981; Eriksen and Larsson, 1981; Eskay et al, 1981; Fukuda et al, 1981; Karten and Brecha, 1980; Lorèn et al, 1980; Münz et al, 1982; Osborne et al, 1981, 1982; Sano et al, 1981; Tornqvist et al, 1981; Yamada et al, 1980, 1981; Kuwayama et al, 1982; unpublished observations). Neuropeptides in most cases are present only within amacrine cells, although there is now good evidence for the presence of peptide-containing interplexiform and perhaps ganglion cells (Brecha, 1983; Brecha et al, 1982B; unpublished observations). Recently, an APP, LRF and FMRF-NH$_2$ immunoreactive retinal centrifugal system has been described in the teleost (Münz et al, 1982; Stell, personal communication). Interestingly, peptide-like substances which are present in the retina are usually localized to one or two morphologically distinct cell types (Brecha, 1983; Karten and Brecha, 1982) (Table 3). Moreover, and perhaps most important, each peptide-containing cell type is different in its morphology and histochemistry from other peptide-containing cell types. These differences in morphology, especially in the arborization pattern of their processes, may be quite striking or very subtle (see below). Recent studies of (A) the localization of SP immunoreactivity in several different vertebrate species and (B) the localization of several peptides in the avian retina clearly demonstrate these general observations and will be discussed below. Overall immunohistochemical studies suggest that each immunohistochemical cell type makes up a distinct and unique population of cells. These morphological observations imply that there is a distinct functional role for each of the peptide-containing cell populations in retinal processing.

A) Distribution of SP immunoreactivity in the vertebrate retina

Recent studies have described the localization of SP immunoreactivity in a variety of vertebrate species (Table 3) (Brecha,

TABLE 3

LOCALIZATION OF SUBSTANCE P-LIKE IMMUNOREACTIVITY IN THE RETINA OF
VARIOUS VERTEBRATES

	GCL	IPL	INL	OPL	# CELL TYPES
-FISH-					
Goldfish (Carassius auratus)	+	3	+		1
Pile Perch (Damanichthys vacca)		1,5	+		1*
Cohoe salmon		1,5	+		1*
Sturgeon poacher		1	+		1
Plainfin midshipman (Porichthys pacifica)		1,5	+		1*
Surfsmelt (Hypomesus pretisus)		5	+		1
Rockfish (Sevastes caurinus)		1,2,4,5	+		1*
Carp		3	+		1
-AMPHIBIANS-					
Xenopus laevis	+	1,2,4,5	+		2*
Toad (Bufo marinus)	+	1,2,3,4,5	+		2*
Frog (Rana pipiens)		3,5	+		1*
Tiger Salamander (Ambysoma tigrinum)		3,5	+		1*
Mudpuppy (Necturus maculosus)		1,5	+		1
-REPTILES-					
Turtle (Chrysemys scripta)		M	+		1*
Lizard (Anolis carolinensis)		3	+		1
Lizard (Uta stansburiana)	+	3	+		1
Lizard (Gecko gecko)		1,3,5	+		1
-BIRDS-					
Pigeon (Columba livia)		3	+		1
Chicken (Gallus domesticus)		3	+		1
-MAMMALS-					
Rat		M	+		1*
Rabbit	+	1,3,5	+	+	3*
Cat	+	3			1
New World monkey (Saimmira sciureus)	+	1,3,5	+		2*
Old World monkey (Macaca nemestrima)	+	1,3,5	+	+	4*
(Macaca facicularis)		3	+	+	1*

*and possibly more cell types
M=multistratified, GCL=ganglion cell layer, IPL=inner plexiform
layer, INL=inner nuclear layer, OPL=outer plexiform layer.

1983; Brecha et al, 1981B, 1982B; Karten and Brecha, 1980; Eskay et
al, 1981; Famiglietti et al, 1980; unpublished observations).
Specific SP immunoreactivity may be present in amacrine, displaced
amacrine, interplexiform and perhaps ganglion cells. These immunoreactive cells and their processes are distributed throughout the
retina and usually their highest densities are within central
retinal regions.

A single, seemingly distinct population of unistratified SP-
containing amacrine cells is present in some species including the

goldfish (Carassius auratus), lizard (Uta stansburiana) and pigeon
(Columba livia) (Brecha et al, 1981B; Karten and Brecha, 1980;
Osborne et al, 1982; unpublished observations) (Figure 1). In these
species, SP-containing cells typically have an ovoid shape, a small
diameter soma, and in most cases, a single primary process which
descends to and ramifies within lamina 3 of the IPL. In each of
these species, SP-containing cells are located at or near the border
of the INL and IPL. There are, however, some difference in the
immunohistochemical patterns observed in these retinas. In goldfish
retina, SP immunoreactive cells are characterized by a medium
caliber primary process which in lizard and pigeon retina, these
cells are characterized by a fine caliber primary process. In the
Uta retina, SP processes are distributed in a broader band within
the IPL than in either the goldfish or pigeon retina. Furthermore,
SP-containing cells in the goldfish and lizard are scattered
throughout the retina and to date no obvious regional differences
have been described. In contrast, SP-containing amacrine cells in
the pigeon are distributed preferentially within peripheral and ventral retinal regions. The SP-containing amacrine cells, in the
pigeon, resemble unistratified cell types depicted by Cajal (1893)
and Boycott and Dowling (1969) from their Golgi and reduced silver
retinal preparations.

    In contrast to the relatively simple SP immunoreactive patterns
observed in the goldfish, Uta, and pigeon retina are the SP immuno-

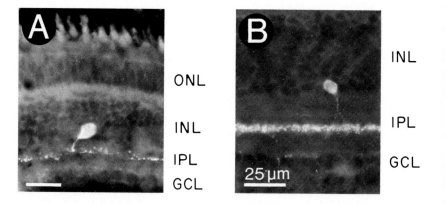

Figure 1. Unistratified SP immunoreactive amacrine cell in (A)
goldfish and (B) Uta lizard retina. These cells usually give rise
to a single process which ramifies in lamina 3 of the IPL.

reactive patterns observed in mudpuppy (Necturus maculosus), bull-frog (Rana catesbeiana), frog (Rana pipiens), toad (Bufo marinus), lizard (Gecko gecko), rabbit, and monkey (Macaca nemestrima, Saimmira sciureus) retinas (Table 3) (Brecha et al, 1982B; Eskay et al, 1981; Famiglietti et al, 1980; unpublished observations) (Figure 2). In these retinas the majority of SP immunoreactivity is distributed in the INL and IPL but it may also be present in the GCL. SP immunoreactivity thus appears to be present in several distinct cell populations in these retinas (vide infra).

In mudpuppy retina, SP immunoreactivity is present in amacrine cells which may have bistratified processes (unpublished observation) (Figure 2A). These SP-containing cells have a round shape and give rise to processes which are distributed predominantly to lami-

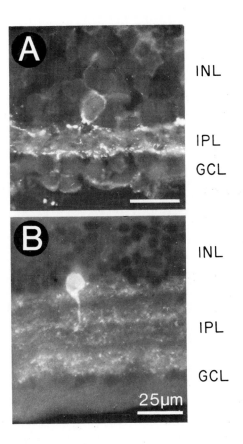

Figure 2. SP-immunoreactive processes and somata in the (A) mud-puppy and (B) Gecko gecko retina. Cells in these retinas give rise to processes which ramify in different lamina of the IPL. Note the differences in SP immunoreactive staining patterns between this figure and figures 1 and 3.

nae 1 and 5 of the IPL. These immunoreactive cells are usually located in the INL at the border of the IPL and are present in all retinal regions. In contrast, in both the bullfrog and toad retina, SP-containing cells are present in the INL and GCL and their processes are distributed in several or all laminae of the IPL (Eskay et al, 1981; unpublished observations). These observations suggest the presence of a minimum of two SP immunoreactive cell populations; amacrine cells and displaced amacrine cells and/or possibly ganglion cells. However, since detailed immunohistochemical studies have not been conducted, it is not possible to suggest the number of distinct SP-containing cell populations which may be present in these retinas. These observations do however, clearly demonstrate that SP immunoreactive cells may have bistratified or multistratified processes.

In the rabbit, as in some other vertebrates, SP immunoreactivity may be present in several distinct retinal cell populations (Table 3). In rabbit retina, SP immunoreactive somata are located in the INL and GCL and the majority of their processes are located in the IPL (Figure 3) (Famiglietti et al, 1980). SP immunoreactive processes are distributed within laminae 1, 3 and most prominently, 5 of the IPL (Figures 3A and 3B). An occasional SP immunoreactive process is also present in the OPL. At least three populations of retinal cells contain SP immunoreactivity. One is located at the border of the INL and IPL and gives rise to a single, stout process which descends to and ramifies within lamina 5 of the IPL (Figure 3A). A second amacrine cell type gives rise to several fine caliber processes which ramify in laminae 1, 3 and 5 of the IPL. Finally, SP-containing cells whose somata are located in the GCL give rise to several primary processes which ramify within lamina 5 of the IPL (Figure 3B). To date, no axon-like process has been observed to be associated with these cells, however, a few scattered SP-containing processes are present in the GAL suggesting the possible existence of SP-containing ganglion cells. This suggestion is supported by a radioimmunoassay study describing SP immunoreactivity in rabbit optic nerve extracts (Unger et al, 1981).

In both the rabbit and Macaca retina, a few immunoreactive processes are also observed in the distal INL and the OPL (Table 3) (Brecha et al, 1982B; Famiglietti et al, 1980). These processes course radially through the INL and upon entering the OPL run tangential to the vitreal surface for a short distance. These immunoreactive processes do not appear to ramify into finer processes within either the INL or OPL (Brecha et al, 1982B). Although the

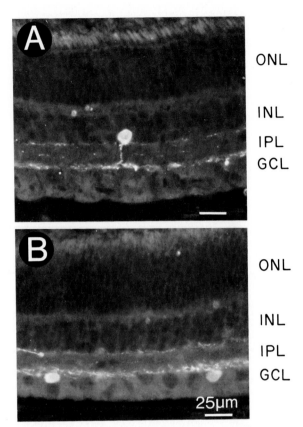

ONL

INL

IPL
GCL

ONL

INL

IPL
GCL

25μm

Figure 3. SP immunoreactivity in the rabbit retina. (A) Unistratified SP immunoreactive amacrine cell. This type of SP-containing
amacrine cell gives rise to a single stout process which ramifies in
lamina 5 of the IPL. Note the laminar distribution of SP-containing
processes in laminae 1, 3 and 5 of the IPL. (B) SP immunoreactivity
in displaced amacrine cells or perhaps ganglion cells. SP-containing cells in the GCL typically give rise to processes which
ramify only in lamina 5 of the IPL.

somata giving rise to these processes have not been identified,

their presence does imply the existence of SP-containing interplexi-

form cells.

Earlier reports of SP biological activity (Winder and Patsalos,

1974) and immunoreactivity (Kanazawa and Jessell, 1976; Reubi and

Jessel, 1978; Unger et al, 1981) in optic nerve extracts and the

presence of SP-containing cells in the GCL of the bullfrog, toad,

rabbit and monkey retina (Brecha et al, 1982B; Eskay et al, 1981;

Famiglietti et al., 1980; unpublished observations) suggests the

existence of SP-containing ganglion cells. This suggestion can be

directly tested by double label experiments using retrograde trans-

port techniques in combination with immunohistochemistry and would provide a final identification and classification of these SP immunoreactive cells.

In conclusion, SP immunoreactivity is distributed in morphologically distinct retinal cell types in every vertebrate species studied to date. SP may be present in amacrine, displaced amacrine, interplexiform and/or ganglion cells. These general patterns of SP immunoreactivity as described above are representative of the patterns of CCK, ENK, GLU, SRIF and VIP immunoreactivity observed in other vertebrate retinas (Brecha, 1983; Brecha et al, 1979, 1980, 1981A, 1982A; Buckerfield et al, 1981; Ericksen and Larsson, 1981; Osborne et al, 1981; Yamada et al, 1980, 1981; Lorèn et al, 1980; unpublished observations).

B) Distribution of neuropeptide-like immunoreactivity in the avian retina

Using the bird retina as a model system, detailed studies of the presence and distribution of peptide-like immunoreactivity have been conducted (Brecha, 1983; Karten and Brecha, 1982; Brecha and Karten, 1983).

The presence of ENK, GLU, NT, SP, SRIF and VIP immunoreactivity by radioimmunoassy within the avian retina has been reported (Brecha et al, 1981A, 1982A; Buckerfield et al, 1981; Eiden et al, 1980; Eskay et al, 1981; Humbert et al, 1979; Reubi and Jessell, 1978) (Table 4). These studies indicate the presence of at least six neuropeptides in the avian retina, which as described below, are present in discrete amacrine cell populations. These studies also indicate that both CCK and TRH immunoreactivities are either absent or very low in the chick retina (Eiden et al, 1980; Eskay et al, 1980).

Immunohistochemical studies have identified six specific neuropeptide-containing amacrine cell populations in the pigeon retina (Brecha and Karten, 1983; Brecha et al, 1979, 1980, 1981A, 1982A; Karten and Brecha, 1980). These studies have clearly established the presence of unistratified SP and multistratified ENK, NT and SRIF immunoreactive cell populations. In addition, preliminary studies have suggested the presence of at least two VIP- and three GLU-containing cell populations. As described below, each of these immunoreactive substances is present in morphologically distinct amacrine cells which differ from one another.

TABLE 4
CONTENT OF VARIOUS NEUROPEPTIDES IN THE AVIAN RETINA

CCK	0.04 ng/retina	chick (1)	
ENK	7.8 ng/retina	chick (1)	
	1.06 fmoles/mg protein	11 day chick embryo (2)	
	0.15 fmoles/mg protein	11 day chick embryo (2)	
GLU	10 pmole/g wet wt.	pigeon (3)	
NT	15.4 fmoles/mg protein	pigeon (4)	
SP	3 fmoles/mg protein	pigeon (5)	
	46 fmoles/mg protein	pigeon	(unpublished)
	25 pg/mg wet wt.	chick	(6)
SRIF	527 fmoles/mg protein	pigeon	(4)
	102 pg/mg wet wt.	chick	(6)
	2.1 ng/mg protein	chick	(7)
TRH	0.1 pg/mg wet wt.	chick	(6)
VIP	0.049 pmoles/mg protein	pigeon	(unpublished)

1 Eiden et al, 1981; 2 Humbert et al, 1979; 3 Brecha et al, 1982A; 4 Brecha et al, 1981A; 5 Reubi and Jessell, 1978; 6 Eskay et al, 1980; 7 Buckerfield et al, 1981.

ENK, NT and SRIF immunoreactivity is present in what appears to be specific populations of multistratified amacrine cells in both the pigeon and chicken retina (Brecha et al, 1979, 1981A; Bucker-field et al, 1981; Tornqvist et al, 1981) (Figure 4). In central retina, ENK-containing multistratified amacrine cells are character-ized by a single process which descends to the border of the IPL before arborizing into several secondary processes. These processes ramify in lamina 1 and give rise to processes which descend to and ramify within lamine 3, 4 and 5 of the IPL.

In pigeon retina, SRIF and NT immunoreactive cells, like the ENK-containing amacrine cells, give rise to a single process which descends to lamina 1 of the IPL before ramifying into several secon-dary processes. Some of these secondary processes then descend to and ramify within laminae 3 and 4 of the IPL. The ENK, SRIF and NT immunoreactive cells measure about 7 µm in diameter, are located in the proximal INL and are distributed in all retinal regions. The density of these immunoreactive cells is the greatest in the red area of the superior retina.

ENK, SRIF and NT immunoreactive amacrine cells are strikingly similar in their appearance (Figure 4). The multistratified cells have similar sized somata which usually give rise to a single

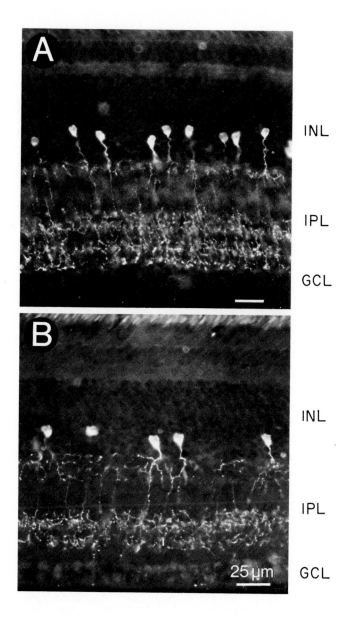

Figure 4. (A) ENK-containing amacrine cells located in the central retina of the pigeon. These cells give rise to multistratified processes which ramify in laminae 1, 3, 4 and 5 of the IPL. (B) NT immunoreactive amacrine cells located in the central retina of the pigeon. These cells give rise to multistratified processes which ramify in laminae 1, 3 and 4 of the IPL. Enkephalin antiserum used for this study was supplied generously by Dr. K.-J. Chang, and neurotensin antisera used in this study was supplied generously by Dr. M. Brown and Mr. J. Koeing.

primary process which descends to and ramifies in lamina 1 of the
IPL. The secondary immunoreactive processes in lamina 1 in turn
give rise to processes which descend to and ramify in more proximal
regions of the IPL. However, on the basis of their histochemistry
it is clear the ENK-, SRIF- and NT-containing amacrine cells consti-
tute separate cell populations. That is, double label immunohistochemical experiments have demonstrated there is not overlap of
staining of each cell type in the same section (Brecha, 1983; Brecha
et al, 1981A; Karten and Brecha, 1982). Furthermore, there are fine
morphological differences in the appearance of these immunoreactive
cell types, especially in the arborization pattern of their processes within the proximal IPL, which also suggests that they belong to
separate populations.

Unistratified SP containing amacrine cells are present in the
pigeon retina (Karten and Brecha, 1980; Osborne et al, 1982). As
described above, these cells give rise to a single process which
arborizes in lamina 3 of the IPL. Interestingly their density is
greatest in peripheral and inferior retinal regions unlike the ENK-,
NT- and SRIF-containing amacrine cells.

In the pigeon retina, VIP immunoreactivity is present within
medium size somata measuring about 12 µm in diameter which are
located at the border of the INL and IPL and in processes which are
present with laminae 1, 3 and 5 of the IPL (Brecha, 1983). These
processes are most prominent in lamina 3 and 5 of the IPL. VIP-
containing amacrine cells typically give rise to a single process
which descends and ramifies in two bands at the border of lamine 2
and 3 and within lamina 5 of the IPL. An occasional VIP-containing
cell has been observed to give rise to processes which ramify in
lamina 1 of the IPL. Whether these cells also give rise to processes which ramify in more proximal regions of the IPL remains to be
investigated. The pigeon retina may thus contain uni-, bi-, and/or
tristatified VIP immunoreactive amacrine cells, although further
studies are needed to establish the exact number of different VIP-
containing amacrine cell types.

GLU immunoreactivity has been reported in both pigeon and
chicken retina (Brecha et al, 1980, 1982A; Kuwayama et al, 1982;
Tornqvist et al, 1981). In the pigeon retina, GLU immunoreactivity
is present in cell bodies located in the INL at the border of the
IPL, and in processes which are most prominent in lamina 1 of the
IPL and in the ora serrata (Brecha and Karten, 1983; Brecha et al,
1980, 1982A; unpublished observations (Figures 5 and 6). In central
retina, the majority of GLU immunoreactive cells have a round shape,

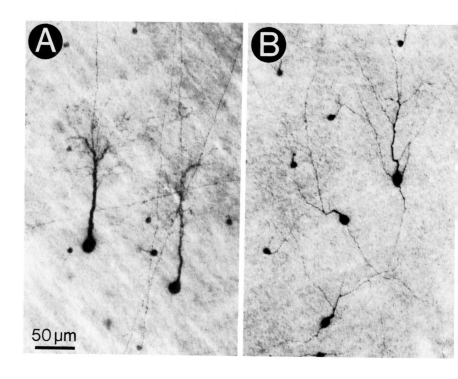

Figure 5. GLU immunoreactivity in the pigeon retina as seen in
retinal whole mount preparations. (A) Medium to large unipolar
cells which are distributed primarily in ventral retinal regions.
(B) Medium sized cells in peripheral retinal regions. Glucagon
antiserum for this study was supplied by Dr. N. Track.

measure about 7 μm in diameter and usually give rise to one, and on
occasion two or three primary processes which arborize in lamina 1
of the IPL. Some of these processes give rise to secondary processes which descend to and arborize within a thin band in lamina 3 of
the IPL. These cells are present in all retinal regions. A second
GLU immunoreactive retinal cell population is located most prominently if not exclusively in ventral retinal regions. These cells
have a round shape and a medium to large somata measuring about 18
μm in diameter (Figure 5A). These cells are characterized by a
single thick primary process which courses tangetial to the vitreal
surface in lamina 1 of the IPL for a short distance before ramifying
into many fine processes which are distributed to laminae 1, 3 and 5
of the IPL. One of these fine processes courses in lamina 1
directly to the edge of the retina where it joins a fascicle of GLU
immunoreactive processes (Figure 6B) which are present next to the
ora serrata. A third population of GLU immunoreactive cells is

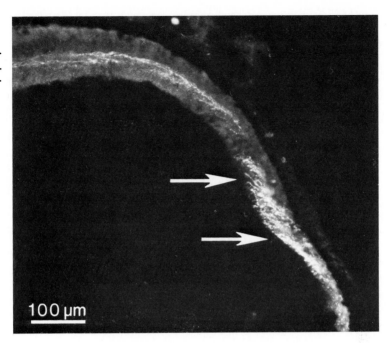

INL
IPL
GCL

100 µm

Figure 6. GLU immunoreactivity in the pigeon retina. Transverse
section of the peripheral retina including the ora serrata. Note
the dense plexus of proceses at the peripheral margin of the retina
in the ora serrata (arrows). Glucagon antiserum for this study was
supplied by Dr. N. Track.

found in peripheral retinal regions. These cells have medium size
somata measuring about 12 µm and two or three primary processes
which ramify in lamina 1 and perhaps deeper lamina of the IPL
(Figure 5B). Some of these processes also join the fascicle of GLU-
containing processes which course through the ora serrata and
encircle the retina. These observations suggest at least 3 types of
GLU-containing cells; the majority of cells in central retinal
regions appear to be uni- and/or bistratified amacrine cells.
However, the medium to large diameter immunoreactive cells located
in ventral and peripheral retinal regions differ slightly from
traditionally described amacrine cells in that their processes
course through the IPL sometimes over several hundred microns to
peripheral retinal regions where they form a fascicle of GLU-containing processes next to the ora serrata.

C) Co-occurrence of neuropeptide-like immunoreactivity with "conventional" transmitters

In addition to peptide immunoreactive amacrine cell populations, other histochemically identified amacrine cells have been identified in the avian retina. These include catecholamine fluorescence, D-aspartate-, Υ-aminobutyric acid (GABA)-, glycine-, choline-, and indoleamine-accumulating, and serotonin-, tyrosine hydroxylase-(TH) and L-glutamate decarboxylase (GAD)-like immunoreactive amacrine cells (Baughman and Bader, 1977; Brecha, 1983; Brecha and Karten, 1983; Ehinger, 1967, 1981; Marshall and Voaden, 1974A, 1974B;d Floren, 1979; Hauschild and Laies, 1973; Oyster et al, 1982; Yazulla and Brecha, 1980; unpublished observations).

A comparison of peptide immunoreactive amacrine cells to choline- and indoleamine-accumulating (Baughman and Bader, 1977; Floren, 1979) and serotonin-like immunoreactive amacrine cells suggest these are separate populations. Choline-accumulating amacrine cells have somata located within the proximal INL and GCL and processes which ramify exclusively in laminae 2 and 4 of the IPL (Baughman and Bader, 1977). Indoleamine-accumulating, indoleamine fluorescence and serotonin-like immunoreactive amacrine cells appear to be identical on the basis of their morphology and are likely to be the same cell type (Floren, 1979; Hauschild and Laties, 1973). These cells have somata in the mid region of the INL and give rise to a single primary process which descends to and ramifies in lamina 1 of the IPL (Figure 7). Processes in lamina 1, in turn give rise to very fine processes which descend to and ramify in lamina 5 of the IPL. Clearly, the morphologies of the choline-accumulating and the serotonin-like immunoreactive amacrine cells are different from the morphologies of the peptide-containing amacrine cells described above, and on this basis it is unlikely that either acetylcholine or serotonin co-occur with any of the retinal neuropeptides described to date.

Dopamine-containing cells in the retina may be recognized using either the Falck-Hillarp histofluorescence technique or antiserum directed to tyrosine hydroxylase, the rate limiting enzyme for the synthesis of dopamine. Catecholamine fluorescent (Ehinger, 1967) and TH immunoreactive (Oyster et al, 1982) amacrine cells give rise to processes which ramify predominantly in lamina 1 as well as at the margins of laminae 2 and 3 and 4 and 5 of the IPL. In peripheral retina, preliminary studies (Oyster et al, 1982) have demonstrated that a large proportion of TH immunoreactive cells are bistratified and their processes are distributed to laminae 1 at the

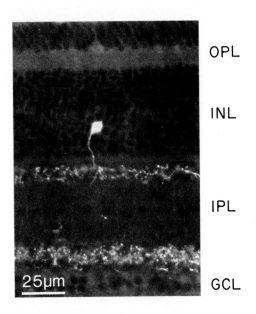

OPL

INL

IPL

GCL

25µm

Figure 7.   Serotonin-like immunoreactivity in the pigeon retina.
Serotonin-like immunoreactivity is distributed in somata which give
rise to bistratified processes which are distributed in laminae 1
and 5 of the IPL.

margin of laminae 2 and 3 of the IPL.   TH-containing cells super-
ficially resemble the GLU and VIP immunoreactive and amacrine cells.
However (a), TH immunoreactivity is not present in the ora serrata
and (b) the number of TH-containing amacrine cells is markedly less
than the number of GLU- and VIP-containing amacrine cells (Karten
and Brecha, 1982). These observations suggest that TH immunoreactivity is not present in every cell that contains either GLU or VIP
immunoreactivity.   It remains possible that TH immunoreactivity is
present in a subset of GLU or VIP immunoreactive amacrine cells.

    GABAergic cells in the retina have been recognized using either
high affinity uptake techniques in combination with autoradiography
or with antiserum directed to L-glutamate decarboxylase, the GABA
synthesizing enzyme.   GAD-like immunoreactivity is present in a
variety of different sized somata distributed throughout the proximal INL and processes which are mainly found in three broad bands in
the IPL best corresponding to laminae 1, 3 and 5.   Whether neuropeptides are present within the GAD-containing or GABA-accumulating
amacrine cells is unknown (Brecha, 1983; Marshall and Voaden, 1974B;
Yazulla and Brecha, 1980).   Finally, no information is available on
the possiblility that neuropeptides are present in D-asparate-

126

and/or glycine-accumulating amacrine cells (Ehinger, 1981; Marshall and Voaden, 1974A).

Overall, these studies suggest that at least in bird retina, peptide immunoreactive amacrine cells are not likely to contain a second peptide and/or "conventional" transmitter substance. Thus, on the basis of histochemical criteria at least twelve distinct populations of amacrine cells have been identified in the pigeon retina (Figure 8).

The histochemical staining patterns observed in these studies suggest possible physiological interactions of amacrine cells in the pigeon retina. For instance, the choline-accumulating amacrine cells whose processes are present in laminae 2 and 4 of the IPL would not be expected to interact with GABA, dopamine, indoleamine and most peptide amacrine cells whose processes do not ramify in these lamina. In contrast, an interaction of several of these amacrine cells systems could be expected in lamina 1 of the IPL. For instance the ENK, NT, SRIF and GLU immunoreactive amacrine cells may interact with one another or with the dopamine, GABA or indoleamine amacrine cells. The possible combinations and interactions are thus immense and further studies are now needed to clarify the synaptic relations of these histochemically identified amacrine cells.

In conclusion, specific neuropeptide-like immunoreactivity is present in at least six amacrine cell populations in the pigeon retina. Other histochemical data indicate that several additional and distinct amacrine cell populations are also present. The existence of these distinct populations suggests that each of the amacrine cell types plays a defined and perhaps unique role in retinal processing.

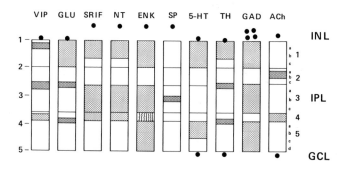

Figure 8. Schematic summary of the distribution of various neuropeptides and transmitter-related substances in the pigeon IPL, indicating the differential distribution of their processes to various laminae of the IPL.

OCCURRENCE OF NEUROPEPTIDES IN THE DEVELOPING CHICKEN RETINA

Recently, preliminary studies have examined the appearance of neuropeptides in the developing chick retina (Brecha et al, 1980; Morgan et al, 1981; unpublished observations) in an effort to gain further insight into their role in retinal function.

Radioimmunoassay studies have described the presence of SRIF, ENK and GLU immunoreactivities in the chick retina a day or two before these peptide-like substances are observed by immunohisto-chemical techniques (Brecha et al, 1980; Morgan et al, 1981; unpub-lished observations). For example, a recent unpublished radio-immunoassay study of GLU immunoreactivity demonstrates that retinal GLU content increases gradually from embryonic day 11 up to hatching, which occurs on about day 21. GLU immunoreactivity peaks at the time of hatching and then decreases to a plateau around day 5 where it remains constant at adult values (Figure 9). A similar sequence is observed for SRIF immunoreactivity as well as other neurotransmitter related substances in the chick retina (Morgan et al, 1981; published observations).

Immunohistochemical studies have also been used to examine the appearance of ENK, SRIF and GLU immunoreactivities in the chick retina (Brecha et al, 1980; Morgan et al, 1981; unpublished observa-tions) and in general, the morphological appearance of peptide-like immunoreactivity in the developing retina has been found to match

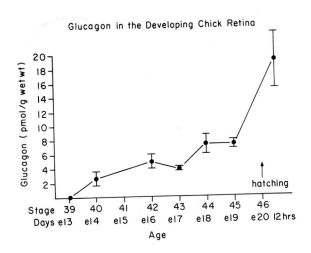

Figure 9. Appearance of GLU-immunoreactivity in the developing chick retina as determined by radioimmunoassay.

the radioimmunoassay time course. However, there are some striking differences in the developmental appearance of immunoreactive staining for these peptides. ENK immunoreactivity is observed in somata, scattered in the INL on embryonic day 13 or 14, but is not present within processes of the IPL until embryonic day 18 or 19 (Brecha et al, 1980; Brecha, 1983). However, within several hours after hatching, ENK immunoreactivity can easily be visualized throughout amacrine cells and their processes and these cells appear to be identical to ENK-containing amacrine cells present in the adult retina. This sequence of events is in marked contrast to that observed for the appearance of GLU immunoreactivity in the chick retina.

GLU-containing somata are first observed about embryonic day 13 or 14, but like the ENK immunoreactive cells seen at embryonic days 18 or 19, do not appear adult-like at this age. However, the GLU-containing amacrine cells appear to develop, at least by the appearance and distribution of peptide-like immunoreactivity, somewhat sooner than the ENK-containing cells.

Interestingly, in neither of these two cases nor in the developing goldfish retina (Brecha et al, 1981B) were the immunoreactive peptides detected in retinal cells which appeared to be migrating, although they were seemingly present in cells which lacked their adult complement of processes. Immunohistochemical studies suggest the earliest time peptide-like substances are present at detectable levels in retinal cells is when the cells begin to give rise to processes within the IPL. However, the earliest age at which these peptides are present is difficult, if not impossible, to determine using current immunohistochemical techniques. Indeed, the radio-immunoassay results suggest that these peptides are present in the retina a day or two before they are detected by immunohisto-chemistry. But, the current studies do clearly demonstrate peptide-like substances (or their precursors) are only present in cells which are likely to be amacrine cells in the developing retina.

PHYSIOLOGICAL STUDIES OF NEUROPEPTIDE SYSTEMS IN THE VERTEBRATE RETINA

The function of neuropeptides in visual processes is unknown, although they undoubtedly make important and critical contributions to retinal functions. This assumption is based upon their presence and widespread distribution in all vertebrate retinas and their localization to specific retinal cell populations. Recent physiological studies also suggest the importance of peptides in visual function. Several of these studies will be briefly reviewed below.

The enkephalin pentapeptides, leu[5]- and met[5]-enkephalin, are reported to influence the release of GABA in the goldfish retina. Previous studies using the teleost retina have demonstrated that GABA is accumulated by selected pyriform amacrine cells (Marc et al, 1980) and released from these cells , by K^+ stimulation, in a Ca^{++} dependent manner (Lam et al, 1980). This K^+ stimulated, Ca^{++} dependent release of GABA is blocked by morphine as well as by met[5]-enkephalin or leu[5]-enkephalin in a dose related manner (Djamgoz et al, 1981). Moreover, the opiate antagonist, naloxone, blocks the suppressive action of met[5]-enkephalin (Figure 10). These data suggest that enkephalin or enkephalin-related peptides have a specific action on GABA-accumulating amacrine cell systems in the teleost retina.

Electrophysiological studies have also provided some evidence for a functional role of enkephalins in the teleost retina (Djamgoz

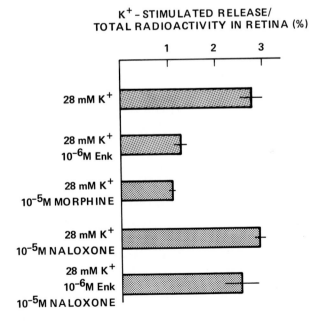

K⁺ - STIMULATED RELEASE/ TOTAL RADIOACTIVITY IN RETINA (%)

Figure 10. Effects of met[5]-enkephalin or leu[5]-enkephalin (Enk), morphine and naloxone on the K^+ stimulated, Ca^{++} dependent release of ^{3}H-GABA from amacrine cells in the goldfish retina. This figure illustrates the inhibition of ^{3}H-GABA release by enkephalins and morphine and the prevention of this effect by the opiate antagonist naloxone. After Djamgoz et al. Reprinted by permission from Nature 292, 620-623. Copyright (c) 1981 Macmillan Journals Limited.

et al, 1981). D-ala^2-met^5-enkephalinamide (DALA), when applied by an atomizer system to an eyecup preparation, at an estimated concentration of 0.1-1.0 μM (a) enhanced spontaneous activity and the light evoked response of ON-center ganglion cells and (b) inhibited the spontaneous activity and the light evoked response of OFF-center ganglion cells. These effects were reversible and prevented by pretreatment of the retina with naloxone. Interestingly, similar but irreversible effects on ganglion cell activity were also observed following morphine application. The physiological actions of the DALA enkephalin analog in the retina is consistent with histochemical observations demonstrating multistratified ENK-containing amacrine cells in the goldfish retina (Stell et al, 1981).

Other studies have also demonstrated peptide effects on retinal cells. For instance application of exogenous substance P has been described to modulate ganglion cell activity in the amphibian and teleost retina (Dick and Miller, 1981; Glickman et al, 1982). Using iontophoretic techniques, substance P or the substance P 4-11 fragment, have been demonstrated to excite all ganglion cells sampled in the mudpuppy retina (Dick and Miller, 1981). In carp retina, in which synthetic substance P was applied by a nebulizer system, substance P was reported to excite most ON- and ON-OFF-center ganglion cells (Glickman et al, 1982). The localization of SP immunoreactivity to amacrine cells in mudpuppy and carp retinas (Figure 3; unpublished observations) and the excitatory action of this substance on ganglion cell discharge is consistent with the idea that substance P is a transmitter in the IPL.

Finally, radioimmunoassay studies suggest that light modulates the level of peptide immunoreactivity. Retinal TRH content, as measured by radioimmunoassay, fluctuates with lighting conditions in the rat (Schaeffer et al, 1977) (Figure 11). TRH levels are highest during light periods and lowest during dark periods. Whether this light/dark difference is related to other circadian rhythms must await a more rigorous analysis. A recent developmental study in the rat has shown that TRH immunoreactivity is not detectable in the retina before the eyes open, is low at eye opening (day 8) and is very high 30 days after eye opening (Martino et al, 1980). At somewhat later time periods, TRH immunoreactivity declines to more intermediate levels characteristic of the adult retina. Interestingly, the appearance of TRH immunoreactivity in the developing rat retina is prevented by maintaining the rat pups in the dark. Both of these experiments (Schaeffer et al, 1977; Martino et al, 1980)

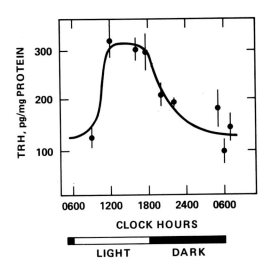

Figure 11. Content of TRH immunoreactivity in the rat retina during a 24 hour period. Retinal content of TRH was several times higher during light periods compared to dark periods. Redrawn; from Schaeffer et al (1977) with permission.

support the notion that the retinal content of TRH immunoreactivity is dependent upon light stimulation. Further support of this notion is provided by a recent morphological study demonstrating light influences VIP immunoreactivity in the rat retina (Eriksen and Larsson, 1981). That is, rat retinas exposed to constant light for 12 days have a greater number of VIP immunoreactive cells and processes than retinas exposed to either a 12 hour light/dark cycle or to constant darkness for 12 days. Interestingly, no changes were observed for SP-, SRIF- and CCK-like immunoreactive staining patterns in rat retinas subjected to these same light/dark treatments.

In conclusion, both release and electrophysiological studies support the proposition that neuropeptides play specific roles, perhaps as neurotransmitters and/or neuromodulators, in the retina. Furthermore, in some cases light appears to have a marked effect on retinal peptide content.

SUMMARY

The presence of several neuropeptide-like substances in the vertebrate retina has been demonstrated by bioassay, immunoassay and immunohistochemistry. Radioimmunoassay and chromatographic studies have demonstrated that these substances are likely to be similar if not identical to previously identified gut and nervous system peptides. Immunohistochemical studies have clearly demonstrated that these immunoreactive peptides are localized to distinct retinal cell types. However, further research, including chromatographic analysis; isolation and characterization of the immunoreactive substances; the identification, characterization and localization of peptide binding sites; and detailed light and electron microscopic analysis of peptide-containing cell populations is needed to clarify the functional role of peptides in the retina.

Studies to date have provided convincing evidence for the existence of distinct neuropeptide-containing retinal cell populations within all vertebrate retinas. Certainly, the localization of these substances to selected retinal cell populations supports the suggestion that peptides play a specific and perhaps unique role in retinal function. This role may be as a neurotransmitter and/or neuromodulator. These substances may thus play a direct role in light activated responsiveness of retinal cells and perhaps they have a role in retinal adaptation to light and dark conditions.

ACKNOWLEDGEMENTS

We would like to express our appreciation to Marianne Cilluffo and Anita Boesman for the help they gave in preparing this review and Dr. Chris Gall for her timely and helpful criticisms. Supported by EY 04067 to N.B., EY 02146 to H.J.K. and AM 17328 to CURE-UCLA - J. Walsh.

REFERENCES

Altshuller, R.A., J.L. Mosinger, D.W. Hoffman and M.H. Parakkal. 1981. Immunocytochemical localization of enkephalin-like immunoreactivity in the retina of the guinea pig. Proc. Natl. Acad. Sci. USA 79; 2398-2400.

Baughman, R.W. and C.R. Bader. 1977. Biochemical chracterization and cellular localization of the cholinergic system in the chicken retina. Brain Res. 138; 469-486.

Boycott, B.B. and J.E. Dowling. 1969. Organization of the primate retina: light microscopy. Phil. Trans. Royal Soc. Lond. B. 255; 109-184.

Brecha, N. 1983. A review of retinal neurotransmitters: Histochemical and biochemical studies. In: Neurochemical Anatomy (Edited by P.C. Emson) New York, Raven Press, in press.

Brecha, N., M. Cilluffo and T. Yamada. 1982A. Localization and characterization of glucagon-like immunoreactivity in the retina. Soc. Neurosci. Abs., 8; 46.

Brecha, N., A. Henderson, I. Floren and H.J. Karten. 1982B. Localization of substance P-like immunoreactivity within the monkey retina. Invest. Ophthalmol. Vis. Sci. 23; 147-153.

Brecha, N.C. and H.J. Karten. 1983. Identification and localization of neuropeptides in the vertebrate retina. In: Brain Peptides (Edited by D. Kreiger, M. Brownstein and J. Martin) New York, Academic Press, in press.

Brecha, N., H.J. Karten and B. Davis. 1980. Localization of neuropeptides, including vasoactive intestinal polypeptide and glucagon within the adult and developing retina. Soc. Neurosci. Abs. 6; 346.

Brecha, N., H.J. Karten and C. Laverack. 1979. Enkephalin-containing amacrine cells in the avian retina: Immunohistochemical localization. Proc. Natl. Acad. Sci. USA 76; 3010-3014.

Brecha, N., H.J. Karten and C. Schenker. 1981A. The localization of neurotensin-like and somatostatin-like immunoreactivity within amacrine cells of the retina. Neuroscience 6; 1329-1340.

Brecha, N., S.C. Sharma and H.J. Karten. 1981B. Localization of substance P-like immunoreactivity in the adult and developing goldfish retina. Neuroscience 6; 2737-2746.

Brownstein, M., A. Arimura, H. Sato, A.V. Schally and J.S. Kizer. 1975. The regional distribution of somatostatin in the rat brain. Endocrinology 96; 1456-1461.

Buckerfield, M., J. Oliver, I.W. Chubb and I.G. Morgan. 1981. Somatostatin-like immunoreactivity in amacrine cells of the chicken retina. Neuroscience 6; 689-695.

Cajal, S.R. 1893. La retine des vertebres. La cellule 9; 17-257.

Dick, E. and R.F. Miller. 1981. Peptides influence retinal ganglion cells. Neurosci. Lett. 26; 131-135.

Djamgoz, M.B.A., W.K. Stell, C.-A. Chin and D.M.K. Lam. 1981. An opiate system in the goldfish retina. Nature 292; 620-623.

Duner, H., U.S. von Euler and B. Pernow. 1954. Catecholamines and substance P in the mammalian eye. Acta. Physiol. Scand. 31; 113-118.

Ehinger, B. 1967. Adrenergic nerves in the avian eye and ciliary ganglion. Z. Zellforsch. 82; 577-588.

Ehinger, B. 1981. [^{3}H]-D-aspartate accumulation in the retina of pigeon, guinea-pig and rabbit. Exp. Eye Res. 33; 381-391.

Eiden, L.E., M.C. Beinfeld and R.L. Eskay. 1980. RIA and HPLC evidence for the presence of methionine enkephalin and cholecystokinin in the neural retina of several vertebrate species. Soc. Neurosci. Abs. 6; 680.

Eriksen, E.F. and L.-I. Larsson. 1981. Neuropeptides in the retina: Evidence for differential topographical localization. Peptides 2; 153-157.

Esch, F., P. Bohlen, N. Lin, R. Benoit, P. Brazeau and R. Guillemin. 1980. Primary structure of ovine hydrothalamic somatostatin-28 and somatostatin-25. Proc. Natl. Acad. Sci. USA. 77; 6827-6831.

Eskay, R.L., R.T. Long and P.M. Iuvone. 1980. Evidence that TRH, somatostatin and substance P are present in neurosecretory elements of the vertebrate retina. Brain Res. 196; 554-559.

Eskay, R.L., J.F. Furness and R.T. Long. 1981. Substance P activity in the bullfrog retina: Localization and identification in several vertebrate species. Science 212; 1049-1051.

Famiglietti Jr., E.V., N.C. Brecha and H.J. Karten. 1980. Neural

134

localization of substance P-like immunoreactivity in rabbit retina. Neurosci. Abs. 6; 212.

Floren, I. 1979. Indoleamine accumulating neurons in the retina of chicken and pigeon. Acta. Ophthamol. Kph. 57; 198-210.

Fukuda, M., Y. Kuwayama, S. Shioska, I. Ishimoto, Y. Shimizu, H. Takagi, S. Inagaki, M. Sakanaka, E. Semba, K. Takatsuki and M. Yohama. 1981. Demonstration of a substance P-like immunoreactivity in retinal cells of the rat. Neurosci. Lett. 23; 239-242.

Glickman, R.D., A.R. Adolph and J.E. Dowling. 1982. Inner plexiform circuits in the carp retina: Effects of cholinergic agonists, GABA, and substance P on the ganglion cells. Brain Res. 234; 81-99.

Hauschild, D.C. and A.M. Laties. 1973. An indoleamine-containing cell in chick retina. Invest. Ophthalmol. 12; 537-540.

Humbert, J., P. Pradelles, C. Gros and F. Dray. 1979. Enkephalin-like products in embryonic chicken retina. Neurosci. Lett. 12; 259-263.

Jackson, I.M.D., J.L. Bolaffi and R. Guillemin. 1980. Presence of immunoreactive β-endorphin and enkephalin-like material in the retina and other tissues of the frog, Rana pipiens. Gen. Comp. Endo. 42; 505-508.

Kanazawa, I. and T. Jessell. 1976. Post mortem changes and regional distribution of substance P in the rat and mouse nervous system. Brain Res. 117; 362-367.

Karten, H.J. and N. Brecha. 1980. Localization of substance P immunoreactivity in amacrine cells of the retina. Nature 283; 87-88.

Karten, H.J. and N. Brecha. 1982. Neuropeptides in the vertebrate retina. In: Neurotransmitter Interaction and Compartmentation (H.F. Bradford, ed.), Plenum Press, New York, in press.

Kobayashi, R.M., M. Brown and W. Vale. 1977. Regional distribution of neurotensin and somatostatin in rat brain. Brain Res. 126; 584-588.

Kuwayama, Y., I. Ishimoto, M. Fukuda, Y. Shimizu, S. Shiosaka, S. Inagaki, E. Senba, M. Sakanaka, H. Takagi, K. Takatsuki, Y. Hara, Y. Kawai and M. Tohyama. 1982. Overall distribution of glucagon-like immunoreactivity in the chicken retina: an immunohistochemical study with flat-mouths. Invest. Ophthal. Vis. Sci. 22; 681-686.

Lam, D.M.K., R.E. Marc. P.V. Sarthy, C.A. Chin, Y.Y.T. Su, C. Brandon and J.-Y. Wu. 1980. Retinal organization: Neurotransmitters as physiological probes. Neurochemistry 1; 183-190.

Loren, I., Tornqvist K. and Alumets, J. 1980. VIP (vasoactive intestinal polypeptide)-immunoreactive neurons in the retina of the rat. Cell Tissue Res. 210; 167-170.

Marc, R.E., W.K. Stell, D. Bok and M.K. Lam. 1978. GABA-ergic pathways in the goldfish retina. J. Comp. Neurol. 182; 221-246.

Marshak, D., J. Reeve, J. Shively and T. Yamada. 1982. Biochemical characterization of retinal somatostatins: sequence of big somatostatin in bovine retina. Soc. Neurosci. Abs. 8; 586.

Marshall, J. and M.J. Voaden. 1974A. A study of [^{3}H] glycine accumulation by the isolated pigeon retina utilizing scintillation radio-autography. Biochem. Soc. Trans. 2; 268-270.

Marshall, J.. and M.J. Voaden. 1974B. An autoradiographic study of the cells accumulating [^{3}]H-γ-aminobutyric acid in the isolated retinae of pigeon and chicken. Invest. Ophthalmol. 13; 602-607.

Martino, E., H. Seo, A. Lernmark and S. Refetoff. 1980. Ontogenetic patterns of thyrotropin-releasing hormone-like material in rat hypothalamus, pancreas, and retina: Selective effect of light deprivation. Proc. Natl. Acad. Sci. USA 77; 4345-4348.

Morgan, I.G., J. Oliver and I.W. Chubb. 1981. The identification and development of amacrine cells containing somatostatin-like immunoreactivity in chicken retina. Soc. Neurosci. Abs. 7; 273.

Mosinger, J.L., D.W. Hoffman and J.C. Gutierrez. 1982. The guinea pig retina contains both met- and leu-enkephalin. Soc. Neurosci. Abs. 8; 45.

Münz, H., B. Claas, W.E. Stumpf and L. Jennes. 1982. Centrifugal innervation of the retina by luteinizing hormone releasing hormone (LHRH)-immunoreactive telencephalic neurons in teleostean fishes. Cell Tissue Res. 222; 313-323.

Osborne, N.N., D.A. Nicholas, A.C. Cuello and G.J. Dockray. 1981. Localization of cholecystokinin immunoreactivity in amacrine cells of the retina. Neurosci. Lett. 26; 31-35.

Osborne, C.W., N.C. Brecha and E.S. Takahashi. 1982. Cholecystokinin and substance P immunoreactivity in retinas of rats, frogs, lizards and chicks. Exp. Eye Res. 34; 639-649.

Oyster, C.W., N.C. Brecha and E.S. Takahashi. 1982. Distribution and morphology of dopaminergic neurons in the retina. Soc. Neurosci. Abs. 8; 586.

Reubi, J.C. and T.M. Jessell. 1978. Distribution of substance P in the pigeon brain. J. Neurochem. 31; 359-361.

Rorstad, O.P., M.K. Senterman, K.M. Hoyte and J. B. Martin. Immuno-reactive and biologically active somatostatin-like material in rat retina. Proc. Natl. Acad. Sci. USA 76; 3019-3023.

Rorstad, O.P., M.K. Senterman, K.M. Hoyte and J.B. Martin. Immuno-reactive and biologically active somatostatin-like material in the human retina. Brain Res. 199; 488-492.

Sano, T., H. Saito, S. Saito, N. Kagawa and K. Hizawa. 1981. Somato-statin-immunoreactive cells in human retina and retinoblastoma. Biomedical Res. 2; 709-713.

Schaeffer, J.M., M.J. Brownstein and J. Axelrod. 1977. Thyrotropin-releasing hormone-like material in the rat retina: changes due to environmental lighting. Proc. Natl. Acad. Sci. USA 74; 3579-3581.

Schally, A.V., W-Y. Huang, R.C.C. Chang, A. Arimura, T.W. Redding, R.P. Millar, M.W. Hunkapiller and L.E. Hood. 1980. Isolation and structure of pro-somatostatin: A putative somatostatin precursor from pig hypothalamus. Proc. Natl. Acad. Sci. USA 77; 4489-4493.

Stell, W.K., K.S. Shohan and N. Brecha. 1981. Enkephalin-immunoreac-tive amacrine cells in the retinas of some teleost fish. Neurosci. Abs. 7; 94.

Tornqvist, K., I. Loren, R. Hakanson and F. Sundler. 1981. Peptide-containing neurons in the chicken retina. Exp. Eye Res. 33; 55-64.

Unger, W.G., J.M. Botler, D.F. Cole, S.R. Bloom and G.P. McGregor. 1981. Substance P, vasoactive intestinal polypeptide (VIP) and somatostatin levels in ocular tissue of normal and sensorily denervated rabbit retinas. Exp. Eye Res. 32; 797-801.

Winder, A.F. and P.N. Patsalos. 1974. Substance P and retinal neurotransmission. Biochem. Soc. Trans. 4; 1260-1261.

Yamada, T., D. Marshak, S. Basinger, J. Walsh, J. Morley and W. Stell. 1980. Somatostatin-like immunoreactivity in the retina. Proc. Natl. Acad. Sci. USA 77; 1691-1695.

Yamada, T., N. Brecha, G. Rosenquist and S. Basinger. 1981. Chole-cystokinin-like immunoreactivity in frog retina: Localization, characterization and biosynthesis. Peptides 2 Suppl. 2; 93-97.

Yazulla, S. and N. Brecha. 1980. Binding and uptake of the GABA analogue, ^{3}H-muscimol, in the retinas of goldfish and chicken. Invest. Ophthalmol. Vis. Sci. 19; 1415-1426.

Evoked Potential Estimates of Infant Visual Development

S. Sokol

The pattern visual evoked cortical potential (VEP) offers a means by which one can study the processing of spatial information in human infants and young children. The VEP is relatively non-invasive, does not depend on extensive motor ability and can be used throughout the entire period of visual development from birth to early childhood without any alterations of the basic paradigm. (For detailed discussions of VEP theory and techniques see Perry & Childers, 1969; Regan, 1972; Sokol, 1976.) The pattern VEP has provided a basis for the study of the development of visual acuity (Marg et al., 1976; Sokol, 1978; DeVries-Khoe and Spekreijse, 1982), contrast sensitivity (Pirchio et al. 1978), spatial-temporal inter-actions (Regan, 1978; Moskowitz and Sokol, 1980), stereopsis (Braddick and Atkinson, 1980; Petrig et al., 1981) and accommodation (Sokol et al., 1982) in both visually normal and abnormal infants and young children. Coincident with VEP studies of infant visual development there has been a number of behavioral studies of visual development primarily based on a forced choice preferential looking paradigm (FPL) (see Dobson, this volume pp. 151-172.)

VISUAL ACUITY

Figure 1 shows VEP estimates of visual acuity for infants up to 7 months of age which have been derived from the amplitude of the VEP. Infant VEP acuity reaches a Snellen "equivalent" of 20/20 (6/6) by 5-6 months of age (Harter & Suitt, 1970; Sokol & Dobson, 1976; Marg et al., 1976; Harter et al. 1977; Sokol, 1978). These results are discrepant with psychophysical data which show that visual acuity at six months is, at best 20/80 and does not reach adult levels until 4-5 years of age (Mayer & Dobson, 1982). This discrepancy may be due, in part, to the different criteria used to

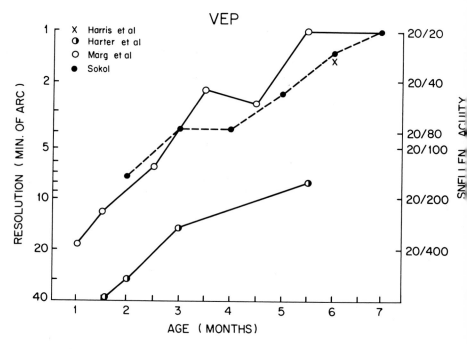

Figure 1. Pattern evoked potential estimates of visual acuity in infants between one and seven months of age. (From Sokol, 1978.)

establish a visual threshold. For example, most behavioral studies of infant acuity are based on the two-alternative forced choice technique and a criterion of 70% correct is usually chosen as threshold. VEP studies, on the other hand, use signal averaging, which increases the signal to noise ratio and improves the "sensitivity" by summing together subthreshold responses. Further, the criterion for VEP threshold has been much lower than behavioral criteria, e.g., extrapolation to 0 vV or comparison of the VEP waveform to a control waveform obtained with a defocused pattern.

In an attempt to reconcile these discrepancies, we have initiated a series of experiments designed to study infant visual function using both VEP and FPL procedures in the same infants with an identical stimulus situation. Figure 2 shows FPL percent correct and VEP waveforms obtained from an 11 week old infant. The stimuli consisted of gratings ranging from 0.3 to 2.5 cycles/degree which were phase reversed at 2 Hz. Recordable VEPs were obtained at 2.5 cycles/degree even though the infant performed at chance in the preferential looking paradigm. Figure 3 shows the proportion of infants between the ages of 8-10 weeks who reached a criterion of

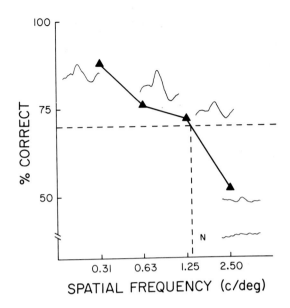

Figure 2. Observer's percent correct in a forced preferential looking paradigm as a function of spatial frequency for an 11 week old infant; vertical dashed line indicates acuity threshold using a 70% criterion. Also shown are pattern evoked potentials obtained on the same day for the four spatial frequencies and for a noise condition. Note that VEPs were obtained at 2.50 cycles/degree which is below the infant's behavioral threshold. Square wave gratings were reversed at 2 Hz.

70% (or above) in a two-alternative forced-choice paradigm using the method of constant stimuli and who elicited VEPs which were significantly different from a noise condition for each of the four spatial frequencies. As spatial frequency increased, there was a sharper decline in the number of infants who elicited evoked potentials that were significantly different from noise.

The results clearly show that VEPs can be obtained from an infant who by behavioral criteria cannot discriminate a patterned from an unpatterned stimulus. These findings emphasize a point made be Teller (1979) that if infants do not prefer a pattern over an unpatterned stimulus it does not necessarily mean that they cannot see it as being different from an unpatterned stimulus. The presence of a VEP demonstrates that information is enough above the noise level of the visual system to be detected at the occipital cortex by the process of computer averaging but that the quality of this information may not be sufficient to elicit discriminable motor responses on the part of the infant.

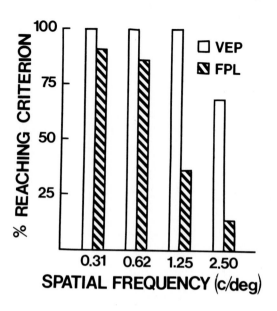

Figure 3. Histogram showing the proportion of infants who: (1) reached 70% criterion in a forced preferential looking paradigm using the method of constant stimuli and (2) produced recordable VEPs, i.e., signals which were significantly different from a noise condition as a function of spatial frequency.

VISUAL ACCOMODATION

A young emmetropic adult is able to focus images clearly over a wide range of distances. This is accomplished by the mechanism of accommodation; as objects move closer the convex power of the lens increases and a focused image is maintained on the retina; as images move away, less power is needed and the lens relaxes. A complete understanding of the development of visual acuity and contrast sensitivity in humans depends, in part, on a knowledge of the infant's ability to accommodate. A number of investigators using retinoscopy (Haynes et al.,1965; Braddick et al.,1979; Banks, 1980) or forced preferential looking techniques (Salapatek et al.,1976; Atkinson et al., 1977) have shown that by 5 months of age infants have a zone of clear vision that encompasses a range of 1 to 6 diopters (100 to 17 cm).

Recent studies with adults have shown that both the amplitude and latency of the VEP can also be used to estimate amplitude of accommodation. Millodot and Newton (1981) found a high correlation between the amplitude of the VEP and the results obtained with a subjective method. Sokol and Moskowitz (1981) measured the latency of the first major positive component (Pl) of the transient pattern reversal VEP and found that latency remained constant as long as the subject was accommodating. When the subject could no longer accommodate and the pattern stimulus appeared blurred, VEP latency increased.

Figure 4 shows the change in VEP latency and the psychophysical estimates of checkerboard blur for adults and one adolescent as a function of increasing minus sphere. The figure shows good agree-

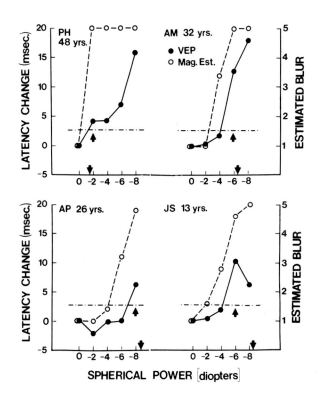

Figure 4. Changes in Pl latency (closed circles) and subjective estimates of blur (open circles) as a function of minus spherical power, in diopters, for 15 minute checks for four subjects. The dash-dot lines indicate the 15% confidence limits (one-tailed) calculated from the data obtained with no lenses (0.0) for all subjects. Upward pointing arrows indicate the first dioptric value where Pl latency was greater than the 95% confidence limits. Downward pointing arrows indicate each subject's amplitude of accommodation as measured with the minus sphere technique (Sloan, 1970). The adults were provided with the following categories to subjectively estimate the magnitude of blur with increasing minus spheres: 1-checks clear; 2-checks initially blurred, but clear without effort; 3-checks initially blurred, but clear with effort; 4-checks initially blurred, only sometimes clear, even with effort; 5-checks always blurred. (From Sokol, Moskowitz and Paul, 1983.)

ment between the onset of subjective blur as measured by clinical and psychophysical techniques and significant increases in VEP latency.

Based on this correlation, we have used the VEP to measure the infant's ability to accommodate (Sokol et al., 1983). Accommodation was stimulated by placing minus lenses of increasing spherical power in front of the infant's eyes. Figure 5 shows records obtained from 2 infants with no lenses and a series of minus lenses of increasing power. Subject AR, tested at 10 weeks with 60 minute checks, showed no change in latency up to 8 diopters. VEPs recorded with 30 minute checks from subject CC at 11 weeks showed little change up to -4 diopters and then an increase in latency at -6 and -8 diopters. Figure 6 shows VEP records from 2 older infants and one adult for 15 minute checks. Infant CT showed no change in latency with -2 and -4 diopters; at -6 diopters, CT's records did not differ from a noise condition. Infant SR, 5 weeks older, showed gradual increases in latency from 2 to 6 diopters. The adult subject with 8.5 diopters

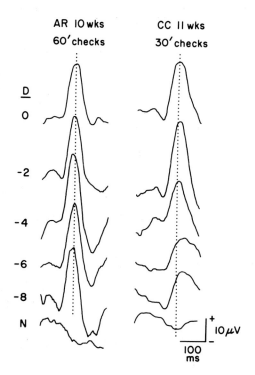

Figure 5. Pattern visual evoked potentials (VEPs) recorded from two infants with increasing amounts of minus sphere. Each subject's age and the check size used to elicit VEPs are shown above the records. D: spherical power in diopters, N: noise condition. Checks reversed at 1.88 Hz. (From Sokol, Moskowitz and Paul, 1983.)

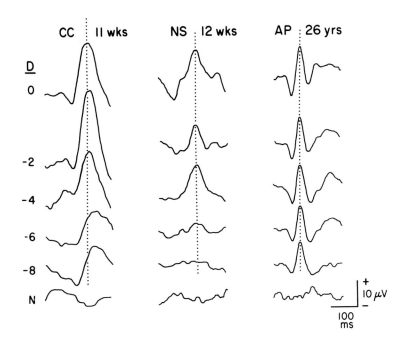

Figure 6. Pattern VEPs obtained from two infants (CC, SR) and one
adult (AP) with increasing amounts of minus sphere.   VEPs were
recorded with 15 minute checks reversing at 1.88 Hz.   The adult
subject had 8.5 diopters of accommodation.   (From Sokol, Moskowitz
and Paul, 1983.)

of accommodation showed no latency change with increasing spherical

power.

Figure 7 shows the proportion of infants who were able to

accommodate as the amount of minus sphere was increased. Infants

whose latencies were less than the 95% confidence limits (which had

been calculated from a no lens condition) were categorized as seeing

the checks clearly; those infants whose values were beyond the 95%

confidence limits were categorized as being unable to accommodate

and therefore saw the checks as blurred.   The figure shows that

infants can accommodate by as much as 9-10 diopters for large

targets (60 minute checks); however, as target size decreases (30

and 15 minute checks), their amplitude of accommodation declines.

One explanation for the infants change in accommodation with

check size is that, like an adult, infants actively change the

optical characteristics of their eye by increasing the amount of

convexity in their lens through contraction of the ciliary muscles

and relaxation of the suspensory ligaments. This would mean, for

example, that when viewing checks through high power concave spheri-

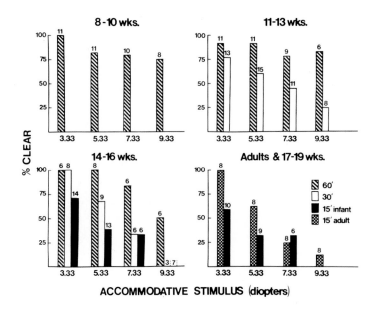

Figure 7. Proportion of infants and adults who maintained clear vision in response to increasing amount of minus sphereical power for 60, 30 and 15 minute checks. The number of subjects treated is shown at the top of each bar. None of the 14-16 week old infants were able to see the 30 and 15 minute checks clearly when -9.33 diopter stimulus was presented. (From Sokol, Moskowitz, and Paul, 1983.)

cal lenses, e.g., minus 9 diopters, the thickness of the infant lens would increase by a relatively large amount in order for the infant to maintain clear vision. But, if infants are capable of a lenticular response of 9-10 diopters for large checks, then they should do equally well when smaller checks are used. However, with smaller checks, their performance is poorer than adults, indicating that they cannot (or will not) exert an accommodative response of this magnitude. An alternative explanation for the results shown in Figure 7 is based on a number of factors that contribute more to an infant's zone of clear vision than to an adult's. These include the infant's poorer visual resolution and contrast sensitivity as compared to the adult and the short axial length of the infant eye.

In conjunction with the difference in the resolving power of the infant and adult eye is the fact that checkerboard patterns were used to record VEPs. The Fourier spectrum of a checkerboard contains, in addition to the fundamental, many lower contrast higher harmonics. For example, a 15 minute checkerboard pattern consists of a fundamental frequency of 2.80 cycles/degree oriented at 45° and

135° as well as a range of harmonics of increasing frequency and decreasing contrast. In the present experiment, the 2.80 cycles/degree component had a contrast of 70% and the harmonic at 30 cycles/degree had a contrast of 4.5% (Kelley, 1976). For 60 minute checks, the frequencies at 70% and 4.5% contrast are 0.71 cycles/degree (the fundamental) and 8 cycles/degree, respectively; and for 30 minute checks the frequencies at 70% and 4.5% contrast are 1.41 cycle/degree and 13 cycle/degree, respectively. Because of the nature of an infant's contrast sensitivity function, (Banks and Salapatek, 1978), it is unlikely that they are responding to the low contrast high spatial frequency components of the checkerboard patterns. For example, the electrophysiologically determined contrast sensitivity function of a 3 month-old-infant (the age at which we obtained data for 3 check sizes) peaks at 1-2 cycle/degree, (Pirchio et al. 1978). We estimate from these data that at 3 months of age an infant would be able to resolve approximately three-quarters of the spatial frequency information available in a 60 minute checkerboard pattern, nearly half of the information in a 30 minute checkerboard pattern but only the fundamental frequency (2.8 cycle/degree) of the 15 minute checks. On the other hand, adults can resolve nearly all of the spatial frequencies present in a 15 minute checkerboard pattern. Thus, the greater ability of the young adults to maintain clear vision with increasing accommodative stimuli (higher power spherical lenses and close distances) is due largely to their higher visual resolution and higher contrast sensitivity as compared to infants.

The depth of focus of the infant's eye also contributes to the results of figure 7. Green et al. (1980) have shown that the infant eye has a greater depth of focus than the adult eye due in part to its shorter axial length. This produces a larger zone of clear vision for the infant than for the adult. For example, the depth of focus values for the 60, 30 and 15 minute checks are 2.48, 1.24 and 0.62 diopters, respectively. Further, if one assumes a resting point of accommodation of two diopters (Howland, 1982), the infant's zone of clear vision for the 3 check sizes without any accommodation would then be 4.48, 3.24 and 2.62 diopters, respectively. Figure 8 shows approximate values of the accommodative effort necessary to see the checks clearly after correcting for the infants' depth of focus. As seen in the figure, little accommodative effort is necessary for any of the check sizes at -3.33 diopters. The maximum amount of effort required for 15 minute checks presented in conjunction with an accommodative stimulus of

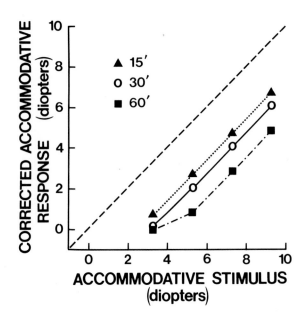

Figure 8. Infants estimated accommodative response after correction for their depth of focus. Accommodative stimuli were minus spherical lenses used at a distance of 75 cm. (From Sokol, Moskowitz and Paul, 1983).

-9.33 diopters is 6.71 diopters. As the histogram of figure 7 shows, none of the infants tested under the -9.33 diopter condition produced recordable responses and only a small proportion of the infants did so when presented with a -7.33 diopter accommodative stimulus. Thus, if one takes into account the infant's poor vision resolution, low contrast sensitivity and large depth of focus, the greatest amount of active accommodation produced by an infant is probably no greater than 5 diopters.

ABNORMAL VISUAL DEVELOPMENT

Abnormalities of the visual system such as strabisums, aniso-metropia, cataracts and ptosis can interfere with the development of visual acuity in the human infant. If the abnormalities are not corrected at an early age amblyopia, which is a reduction in visual acuity in one or both eyes not correctable by optical means can occur. In amblyopia, the amplitude of the pattern VEP is reduced, particularly for checks smaller than 30 minutes of arc (see Figure 9) (Spekreijse et al., 1972; Arden, 1973; Sokol and Bloom, 1973; Arden et al., 1974; Sokol & Shatterian, 1976; Sokol, 1977, 1980). In

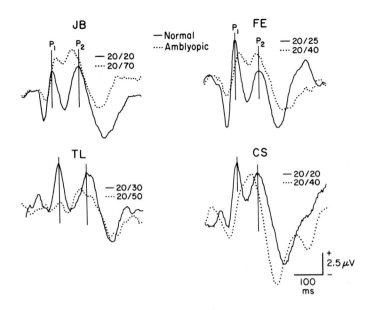

Figure 9. Pattern reversal visual evoked potentials obtained from four amblyopic children. VEPs were recorded with 15 minute checks which phase reversed at 2 Hz.

addition, figure 10 also shows that the latency of the VEP is affected in amblyopia. For example, the records show that P1 latency is slightly longer in the amblyopic eye than in the normal eye, while P2 is shorter in the amblyopic eye, an effect opposite to that found in demyelinating lesions of the optic nerve (Halliday et al. 1972). One possible explanation for a shorter latency in amblyopia is based on the fact that latency varies as a function of spatial frequency. Low spatial frequencies elicit VEPs with shorter latencies than high spatial frequencies (Parker & Salzen, 1977a, b). If one assumes that amblyopia is due to the drop-out of high spatial frequency mechanisms, then shorter P2 latencies in the amblyopic eye may be a reflection of the electrical activity of the remaining middle and low spatial frequency mechanisms.

In addition to the value of the VEP in the detection of amblyopia, it is also useful in monitoring the treatment of amblyopia. Figure 10 shows VEPs obtained from a 5 year old boy with strabismic amblyopia. When the patient was first seen, the amplitude of the VEP recorded from the amblyopic eye was reduced (lower record of figure 10a). Following 3 weeks of full time occlusion of the normal fellow eye the amplitude of the VEP increased concomitant with an

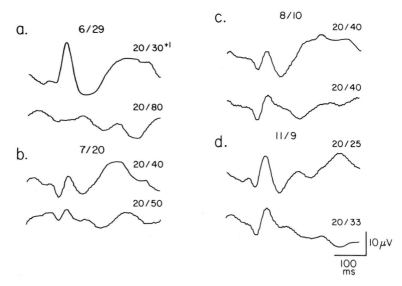

Figure 10.   Pattern VEPs recorded from a 5 year-old strabismic amblyopic before and during occlusion therapy.   The patient's line Snellen acuity is shown next to each record.   Upper record of each pair is the normal eye; lower record, the amblyopic eye.   (From Wilcox and Sokol, 1980).

improvement of acuity to 20/50 (lower record, 10b).   The VEP amplitude in the amblyopic eye continued to improve and reflect nearly equal acuities (10,c d).

SUMMARY

The pattern VEP can be used to study the maturation of the sensory aspects of infants visual system and to measure the changes in visual acuity, contrast sensitivity, accommodation and binocularity as a function of age.   The VEP can also be used to detect visual abnormalities in young children with eye disorders.   The pattern VEP reflects information that has traveled only as far as the occipital cortex and therefore does not represent the final outcome of visual information processing, namely behavior. Accordingly, one should be aware that there may be occasions when the evoked potentials and subjective experience are not correlated.

REFERENCES

Arden, G.B. 1973. The visual evoked response in ophthalmology.
    Proc. Roy. Soc. Med. 66; 1037-1043.
Arden, G.D. and W.M. Barnard and A.S. Mushin. 1974. Visually evoked
    responses in amblyopia. Br. J. Ophthal. 58; 183-192.
Atkinson, J., O. Braddick and K. Moar. 1977b. Development of con-
    trast sensitivity over the first 3 months of life in the human
    infant. Vision Res. 17; 1037-1044.
Banks, M.S. 1980. The development of visual accommodation during
    early infancy. Child Dev. 51; 646-666.
Banks, M.S. and P. Salapatek. 1978. Acuity and contrast sensitivity
    in 1-, 2- and 3-month-old human infants. Invest. Ophthalmol.
    Vis. Sci. 17; 361-365.
Braddick, O. and J. Atkinson. 1980. Cortical binocularity in in-
    fants. Nature 288; 363-365.
Braddick, O., J. Atkinson, J. French and H.C. Howland. 1979. A
    photorefraction study of infant accommodation. Vision Res. 19;
    1319-1330.
DeVries-Khoe, L.H. and H. Spekreijse. 1982. Maturation of luminance
    and pattern EPs in man. In: G. Niemeyer and Ch. Huber (Eds.),
    Docum. Ophthal, Proc. Series, Vol. 31. Junk, The Hague, 461-
    475.
Green, D.G., M.K. Powers, M.S. Banks. 1980. Depth of focus, eye
    size and visual acuity. Vision Res. 20; 827-835.
Halliday, A.N., W.I. McDonald and J. Mushin. 1972. Delayed visual
    evoked response in optic neuritis. Lancet 1; 982-985.
Harris, L., J. Atkinson and O. Braddick. 1976. Visual contrast
    sensitivity of a 6-month-old infant measured by the evoked
    potential. Nature, Lond. 264; 570-571.
Harter, M.R., F.K. Deaton and J.V. Odom. Maturation of evoked
    potentials and visual preference in 6-45 day old infants:
    effects of check size, visual acuity and refractive error.
    Electroenceph. Clin. Neurophysiol. 42; 595-607.
Harter, M.R. and C.D. Suitt. 1970. Visually evoked cortical
    responses and pattern vision in the infant: A longitudinal
    study. Psychon. Sci. 18; 235-237.
Haynes, H., B.L. White and R. Held. 1965. Visual accommodation in
    human infants. Science 148; 528-530.
Howland, H.C. 1982. Personal communication.
Kelly, D.H. 1976. Pattern detection and the two-dimensional Fourier
    transform: Flickering checkerboards and chromatic mechanisms.
    Vision Res. 16; 277-287.
Marg, E., D.N. Freeman, P. Peltzman and P.J. Goldstein. 1976. Visual
    acuity development in human infants: Evoked potential measure-
    ments. Invest. Ophthalmol. 15; 150-153.
Mayer, D.L. and V. Dobson. 1982. Visual acuity development in
    infants and young children, as assessed by operant preferential
    looking. Vision Res. 22; 1141-1152.
Millodot, M. and I. Newton. VEP measurement of the amplitude of
    accommodation. Br. J. Ophthal. 65; 294-298.
Moskowitz, A. and S. Sokol. 1980. Spatial and temporal interaction
    of pattern-evoked cortical potentials in human infants. Vision
    Res. 20; 699-707.
Parker, D.M. and E.A. Slazen. 1977a. Latency changes in the human
    visual evoked response to sinusoidal gratings.
Parker, D.N. and E.A. Salzen 1977b. The spatial selectively of
    early and late waves within the human visual evoked responses.
    Perception, 6; 85-95.
Perry, N.W. Jr. and D.G. Childers. 1969. The Human Visual Evoked
    Response. Springfield, Charles C. Thomas.

Persson, H.E. and P. Wanger. 1982. Pattern-reversal electro-retinograms in squint amblyopia, artificial anisometropia and simulated eccentric fixation. Acta Ophthalmol. 60; 123-132.

Petrig, B., B. Julesz, W. Kropfl, G. Baumgartner and M. Anliker. 1981. Development of stereopsis and cortical binocularity in humans infants: Electrophysiological Evidence. Science, 213; 1402-1405.

Pirchio, M., D. Spinelli, A. Fiorentini and L. Maffei. 1978. Infant contrast sensitivity evaluated by evoked potentials. Brain Res. 141; 179-184.

Regan, D. 1972. Evoked Potentials in Psychology, Sensory Physiology and Clinical Medicine. London, Chapman and Hall.

Regan, D. 1978. Assessment of visual acuity by evoked potential recording: Ambiguity caused by temporal dependence of spatial frequency selectivity. Vision Res. 18; 439-443.

Salapatek, P., A.G. Bechtold and E.W. Bushnell. 1976. Infant visual acuity as a function of viewing distance. Child Dev. 47; 860-863.

Sokol, S. 1976. Visually evoked potentials: Theory, techniques and clinical applications. Survey of Ophthalmology, 21; 18-44.

Sokol, S. 1977. Visual evoked potentials to checkerboard pattern stimuli in strabismic amblyopia. In: Visual Evoked Potentials in Man: New Developments (Edited by Desmedt, J.E.) Clarendon Press, Oxford pp. 410-417.

Sokol, S. 1978. Measurement of infant visual acuity from pattern reversal evoked potentials. Vision Res. 18; 33-39.

Sokol, S. 1980. Pattern visual evoked potentials: Their use in pediatriic ophthalmology. In: Electrophysiology and Psychophysics: Their Use in Ophthalmic Diagnosis. (Edited by Sokol, S.) International Ophthalmology Clinics 20; 251-268.

Sokol, S., and B. Bloom. 1973. Visually evoked cortical potentials of amblyopes to a spatially alternating stimuli. Invest. Ophthalmol. 12; 936-939.

Sokol, S. and V. Dobson. 1976. Pattern reversal visually evoked potentials in infants. Invest. Ophthalmol. 15; 58-62. Latency of the pattern evoked potential. Vision Res. 21; 1279-1286.

Sokol, S., A. Moskowitz and A. Paul. 1983. Evoked potential estimates of visual accommodation in infants. Vision Res. (in press).

Sokol, S. and E.T. Shaterian. 1976. The pattern evoked cortical potential in amblyopia as an index of visual function. In: Orthoptics: Past, Present and Future (Edited by Moore, S., Mein, J. and Stockbridge, L) Transactions of the Third International Orthopic Congress. Miami Symposia Specialists, pp. 59-67.

Spekrijse, H., L.H. Khoe and L.H. van der Tweel. 1972. A case of amblyopia; electrophysiology and psychophysics of luminance and contrast. In: The visual System Neurophysiology, Biophysics and their Clinical Application. Recent Advances in Experimental Biology and Medicine. (Edited by Arden, G.G) Vol. 24, New York, Plenum Press, pp. 141-156.

Teller, D.Y. 1979. The forced-choice preferential looking procedure: A psychophysical technique for use with human infants. Infant Behavior and Development 2; 135-153.

Wilcox, L.M. and S. Sokol. 1980. Changes in the binocular fixation patterns and the visually evoked potential in the treatment of estropia with amblyopia. Ophthalmology, 87; 1273-1281.

Preferential Looking Measures of Visual Acuity in Infants and Young Children

V. Dobson

I. HISTORICAL PERSPECTIVE

All preferential looking procedures are based on the observation, originally noted by Berlyne (1958) and Fantz (1958), that young infants stare more at a pattern than at a blank field. Following up on this observation, Fantz developed a procedure, known as preferential looking (PL), that has allowed researchers to study the visual abilities of the young infant.

In preferential looking, an infant is shown two stimuli. An adult observer, who is looking through a peephole at the infant, watches to see if the infant shows some sort of preferential fixation of one of the stimuli. If, with repeated presentations, the infant continues to show more fixation of one of the two stimuli, regardless of where this stimulus is located with respect to the other stimulus, one can conclude that the infant can discriminate between the two stimuli.

II. PROCEDURES

Young infants. The first use of the preferential looking procedure for the measurement of visual acuity was by Fantz et al., (1962). These researchers tested infants between 2 weeks and 5-1/2 months of age. For testing, each infant was seated in an infant seat and presented with two trials of each of four or five acuity gratings composed of black-and-white stripes. On each trial an acuity grating was paired with a gray homogeneous field of the same size that was matched to the grating in space-average luminance. An adult observer recorded which of the two stimuli the infant looked at first, the total time the infant looked at each stimulus, and the number of times the infant re-fixated each stimulus during a 20-sec. trial. Each infant was shown each grating twice--once with the grating on the left and once with the grating on the right. Since each infant was shown four or five grating frequencies (stripe widths), the total number of trials for each infant was 8 or 10. To determine how acuity changes as a function of age, Fantz and his coworkers combined the data of all infants of the same age and estimated acuity as the grating frequency fixated preferentially by 75 percent or more of infants of that age. Fantz et al.'s results indicated that acuity increased from 0.75 cy/deg (20/800[1]) at 2 weeks to 8.6 cy/deg (20/70) at 5-1/2 months.

In the ten years between Fantz et al.'s study and the early 1970's, little work was done on the behavioral measurement of visual acuity in infants. In 1974, however, Teller et al., published a paper which was to be the first of a rapidly increasing number of papers on infant acuity. In this paper, Teller et al. focused on acuity measures of individual infants using a modified version of Fantz' preferential looking procedure. Teller termed her version of the preferential looking procedure, forced-choice preferential looking (FPL), and it differs from Fantz' version in at least two important ways. First, in FPL, the adult observer does not know whether the acuity grating is on the left or the right side of the screen on each trial. The observer's task is to use the infant's looking behavior to determine the position of the grating. Thus, on each trial, the observer must say whether the grating is on the left or right, and the observer's response is scored as correct or incorrect. This makes the FPL procedure similar to standard forced-choice procedures used in adult psychophysics, and eliminates any possibility that the observer is unconsciously biasing the results by knowing the location and/or the spatial frequency of the acuity grating (see Teller, 1979, for a more complete description of FPL).

A second difference between FPL and the earlier preferential looking procedure is that each infant is shown each grating frequency many times (usually at least 20). This means that enough trials are obtained from an individual infant to provide an acuity estimate for that infant. Typically, a psychometric function such as that shown in Figure 1 is plotted for each infant and acuity is estimated as the grating frequency that would produce an observer's percent correct of 75 percent.

Figure 2 shows infant acuity data obtained in the last ten years with PL and FPL procedures, as well as some of the original PL

---

[1]Based on the convention that grating acuity of 30 cy/deg is equivalent to 20/20 Snellen acuity.

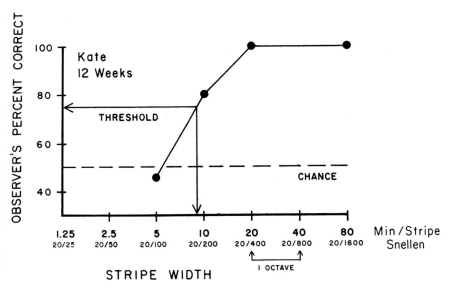

Figure 1. Psychometric function for an infant tested with the forced-choice preferential looking procedure. Observer's percent correct is plotted for the four stripe widths used during testing. Acuity threshold (arrow) is estimated at the stripe width (approximately 10 min. of visual angle) that produced 75 percent correct by the observer. Data points for the three smallest stripe widths are based on 20 trials per stripe width; for the largest stripe width, the data point is based on 30 trials. (Reprinted with permission from Dobson, 1980.)

acuity data of Fantz et al. (1962). It is striking that the more recent data show considerable agreement both among studies and with Fantz et al.'s original results concerning the development of acuity during the first six postnatal months. These results suggest that we are well on the way to developing acuity norms for infants in the 2-week to 6-month age range.

Older infants and toddlers. While it is certainly useful to have a behavioral measure of visual acuity for infants less than 6 months of age, most clinicians would also find it very useful to have a measure of visual acuity for children in the 6-month to 3-year age range. Figure 3 shows the results of a sample of the published studies that have used behavioral techniques to measure visual acuity in children between 2 weeks and 5 years of age. It is clear that there are many more studies that have studied visual acuity before 6 months and after 3 years than have examined acuity between these two ages.

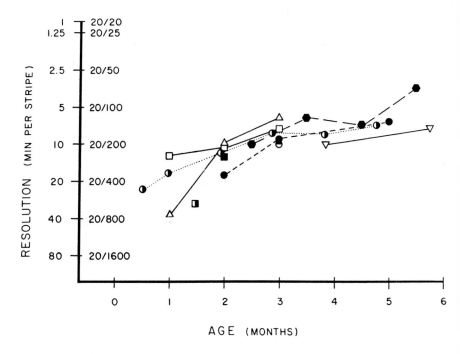

Figure 2. Estimates of visual acuity in infants less than 6 months of age obtained using various versions of the preferential looking technique. Studies shown tested more than 1 infant at each age and used a stimulus luminance of 1.0 log cd/m^2 or greater. ◖- Allen (1979); △ - Atkinson et al., (1977a), Atkinson (1978), and Atkinson (personal communication); ■ - Banks and Salapatek (1976); □ - Banks and Salapatek (1978); ◓ - Dobson et al., (1978); ◆ - Fantz et al., (1962); ▽ - Gwiazda et al., (1978); ▣ - Salapatek et al., (1976); ● - Teller et al., (1974). We have rescored the data of Fantz et al., interpolating between stripe widths used, to estimate the stripe width preferentially fixated by 75 percent of infants tested (Reprinted with permission from Dobson, 1980.)

What are the difficulties involved in testing children between 6 months and 3 years and what methods have been developed to overcome these difficulties? Undoubtedly, the main problems with testing toddlers are their short attention span and their unwillingness to sit still and look at trial after trial of black-and-white stripes. To try to overcome these problems, several researchers have modified the PL procedure to make it more interesting for older infants and toddlers. Atkinson and Braddick (1979) presented acuity stimuli on a bright CRT screen in a dimly illuminated room and obtained acuity estimates from infants up to 9 months. Gwiazda et al., (1978, 1980) tested infants in a room that was totally dark except for the two stimulus screens and were successful at testing

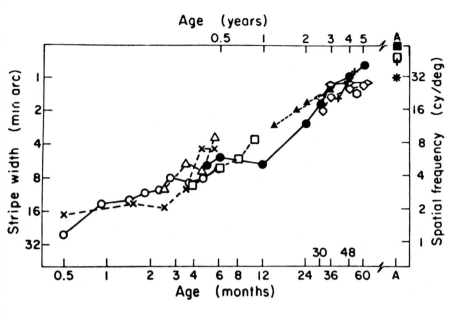

Figure 3. Estimates of acuity in children 2 weeks to 5 years of age obtained using behavioral measures of acuity. For children, the data shown are from: X - Fantz et al. (1962), optokinetic nystagmus; △- Fantz et al. (1962), PL; O- Allen (1979), PL; □- Gwiazda et al. (1978), PL; ●- Mayer and Dobson (1982), OPL; ▲- Gwiazda et al. (1981), operant; +- Atkinson et al. (1981), preferential running; ♀- Lippmann (1971), "E" test; ◇- Woodruff (1972), STYCAR, Allen Test at 30.5 months; ⬭- Roberts and Ludford (1977), Snellen or "E" test. For adults the data are from: +- Atkinson et al. (1981); ■- Mayer and Dobson (1982), forced-choice procedure; ◻- Mayer and Dobson (1982), yes-no procedure. The * indicates the nominal adult Snellen acuity of 20/20. When acuity and age are plotted on log axes, there appears to be a linear improvement in acuity between 2 weeks and 5 years of age (Modified and reprinted with permission from Mayer and Dobson, 1982.)

infants up to 12 months of age. Thus, it is possible to extend the age range over which PL procedures are useful by increasing stimulus salience and decreasing extraneous distractions in the room.

To extend the usefulness of PL procedures beyond infancy, however, it appears to be necessary to add some sort of reinforcement to the procedure, to reward the child for looking at the acuity stimulus and remaining in the test situation. The technique we use to test older infants and toddlers is called operant preferential looking (OPL) (Mayer and Dobson, 1980). The OPL procedure is similar to Teller's FPL procedure in that the observer, who does not know the location of the acuity grating, makes a forced-choice judgement concerning the left-right position of the stimulus on each trial. However, in the OPL procedure the child is taught that if he or she indicates the position of the acuity grating to the observer, either by looking at it or pointing to it, an animated toy located adjacent to the acuity grating will be activated. During testing, the actual toy used (monkey, rabbit, bear, etc.) can be changed as many as four times during the test session, to maintain the child's interest in the procedure. Figure 3 shows data obtained from infants, toddlers, and preschool children tested with the OPL technique (Mayer and Dobson, 1982). Clearly, the OPL procedure has increased the age range over which PL techniques can be used to measure acuity in children. Nevertheless, there is one age group that remains very difficult to test with the OPL procedure--the 1-1/2-year-olds. Most of these children do not stay interested enough in the procedure to learn the association between looking at the acuity grating and activation of the toy animal (Mayer and Dobson, 1982).

Birch et al. (1980) have devised a modification of the PL procedure that has had considerable success with children in the 1- to 2- year old range (Birch, personal communication). In their procedure, the child is taught that if he or she presses on the grating stimulus, a Cheerio will drop into a reinforcement cup below the grating. Thus, the procedure provides the child with enough activity to keep him or her interested in the test procedure for the time required to obtain an estimate of the child's acuity. Preliminary data from Gwiazda et al. (1981) suggest that children in the one- to two-year-old range who are tested with the procedure show better acuity than children in this age range who are tested with the OPL procedure (see Figure 3). For children older than 24 months, there is good agreement between the results of the two procedures.

Finally, Atkinson et al. (1981) have devised a third method for adding reinforcement to the preferential looking procedure. In their procedure, the child is positioned at the end of a barrier. At a distance of 1 to 3 meters from the child, a cube containing a vertical grating is placed on one side of the barrier and a cube containing a horizontal grating is placed on the other side of the barrier. The child is taught that each time he or she runs to the grating of the correct orientation (vertical for some children and horizontal for other children), he or she will find food or toys under the cube. To date, this procedure has been used only with 3- to 5-year old children. As shown in Figure 3, the data reported for this age range are quite similar to the data obtained by Mayer and

Dobson (1982) with the OPL procedure for children in the same age
range.

In summary, the modification of PL procedures for use with
children older than 6- to 12-months of age has occurred only very
recently. There is a considerable need for further refinement of
these techniques and for more extensive studies of normative acuity
values for toddlers.

III. PARAMETERS THAT AFFECT VISUAL ACUITY IN INFANTS

There are many parameters that affect visual acuity in adults.
These include luminance, optical defocus, retinal location of the
stimulus, whether testing was conducted monocularly or binocularly,
the spatial nature of the stimulus (i.e. whether the target was
designed to test detection, recognition, resolution, or localization
acuity), and many other factors (see Riggs, 1965; Committee on
Vision, 1980). To date, however, very few studies have examined the
effects of any of these parameters on preferential looking measures
of acuity, and in those that have, only very young infants were
tested.

Luminance. In adults, numerous studies have shown that when
stimulus luminance is less than about 1.0 log cd/m^2, a decrease in
luminance produces a reduction in visual acuity. On the other hand,
increases in stimulus luminance above about 1.0 log cd/m^2 produce
very little improvement in acuity.

The data shown in Figure 2 suggest that for young infants, too,
variations in luminance in the mid- to high-photopic range may have
little effect on acuity. That is, despite the fact that the
luminance values of the stimuli used in the studies whose results
are shown in Figure 2 ranged from 1.2 to 1.7 log cd/m^2, there is
striking agreement across studies as to the acuity values obtained
at each age.

Further evidence that variations in luminance have little
effect on acuity in young infants comes from a study that we conducted on 2-month olds (Dobson et al., 1983). Each infant's acuity
was measured at 2 to 5 luminance levels using the FPL procedure.
The results of this study are shown in Figure 4, along with data
from five adult subjects tested in the same apparatus and two
infants whose visual evoked potential (VEP) acuity was measured by
Fiorentini et al. (1980), and a line indicating classical data on
acuity vs luminance obtained by Shlaer (1937) from two adult
subjects. These data suggest that for 2-month-olds, as for adults,

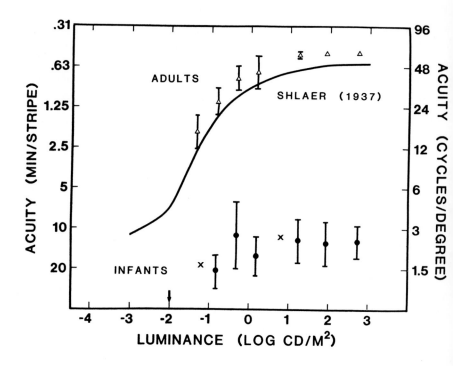

Figure 4. Visual acuity as a function of luminance for 2-month-old infants (filled circles) and adults (open triangles) tested by Dobson, Salem, and Carson (in press). Bars indicate +1 standard deviation. The data from the adults agree well with Shlaer's (1937) classic data on luminance vs. acuity, and the data from the infants agree well with VEP data of Fiorentini et al. (1980) from two infants tested at two luminance levels. For 2-month-old infants, as for adults, acuity is relatively insensitive to variations in luminance above approximately 1.0 log cd/m^2. (Reprinted with permission from Dobson et al., Investigative Ophthalmology and Visual Science, 1983.)

changes in stimulus luminance above about 1.0 log cd/m^2 have little, if any, effect on acuity. Unfortunately, our test procedure made it impossible to test infants at luminances below -0.8 log cd/m^2, so we do not know the extent to which decreases in luminance below 1.0 log cd/m^2 produce a reduction in infants' acuity.

In summary, it appears that variations in luminance in the mid to high photopic range have little influence on acuity in young infants. Although research is needed to study the effects of varia-tions in luminance at lower levels, and the effects of luminance variations on acuity in older infants and toddlers, the results do data suggest that clinicians interested in testing acuity in very young infants do not need to worry about precise control of luminance, as long as luminance is kept above 1.0 log cd/m^2.

Optical defocus. Campbell (1957) showed that adults have a depth of focus of ± 0.43 diopter, which means that even a small amount of optical blurring can reduce an adult's acuity. On the other hand, very young infants have been predicted to have a depth of focus of about ± 1 diopter, due largely to their poor visual acuity (Green et al., 1980). This suggests that young infants would be less affected than adults by optical blur.

We measured the effect of plano, -14, -3, +6, and +14 diopter lenses on visual acuity in 6-week-old infants and as shown in Figure 5, we found that the reduction in acuity shown by the infants was less than that shown by adults wearing lenses of the same power (Powers and Dobson, 1982).[2] These results are interesting in that they suggest that the only 6-week-old infants whose vision would be improved with glasses are those with fairly large refractive errors. However, they are of little practical importance to the clinician since the infants in the study were very young. Given the improvement in acuity that occurs during the first three years of life, it is probable that the acuity of older infants and toddlers would be affected much more by optical defocus than was the acuity of the 6-week-olds. A more extensive discussion of the effects of defocus of VEP acuity in infants can be found in the chapter by Sokol in this volume.

Astigmatism. A number of researchers have shown that a high proportion of infants are astigmatic (Santonastaso, 1930; Mohindra et al., 1978; Howland et al., 1978; Ingram and Barr, 1979; Fulton et al., 1980). Therefore, it would be of interest to know the extent to which astigmatism affects an infant's visual acuity.

Teller et al. (1978) examined acuity for vertical and horizontal gratings in an infant who had a refractive error of -0.50 + 2.5 x 90 O.D. and -1.0 + 2.5 x 90 O.S. At four and five months of

---

[2]It should be noted that the differences between adults and infants in the left-hand-portion of Figure 5 could be due to differences in the accommodative ability of infants and adults. If the accommodative range of infants is larger than that of adults, the addition of minus lenses should have less effect on their acuity than it would for adults. Resolution of this issue awaits the measurement of the infant's full accommodative range. The differences in the degree of acuity reduction produced by the addition of plus lenses (the right-hand portion of the graph) cannot be the result of differences in accommodation, since it is not possible to accommodate to focus a stimulus that is imaged in front of the retina. Therefore, differences between infants and adults in this portion of the curve are probably due to differences in the effects of optical defocus.

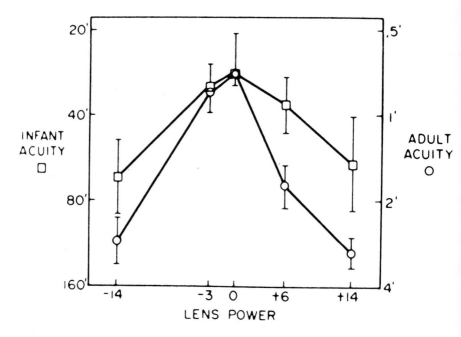

Figure 5. Relative change in acuity with lens power. Squares: mean acuity of 6-week-old infants. Circles: mean acuity of adults. Left ordinate: infant acuity; right ordinate: adult acuity. Curves have been shifted vertically to coincide at plano lens power. Abscissa: lens power in diopters. Bars are + 2 standard errors of the mean. Ten adults and ten infants were tested. (Reprinted with permission from Powers and Dobson, 1982.)

age the infant was tested without optical correction and showed considerably better acuity for vertical than for horizontal gratings. When she was retested at six months she wore optical correction during testing and showed no difference in acuity for the two grating orientations. These results indicate that astigmatism can affect visual acuity in infants less than six months of age and suggest that optical correction can improve an astigmatic infant's acuity.

These results are supported by the results of studies by Held and his colleagues (Held et al., 1977; Held, 1978), in which astigmatic infants were presented with a vertical and horizontal grating simultaneously, and a PL procedure was used to determine whether the infant showed preferential fixation of one of the orientations. These researchers found that for gratings above and below acuity threshold, astigmatic infants showed no preference for vertical vs. horizontal stimuli. However, when the gratings were near the expected acuity threshold, infants with mixed astigmatism who had a myopic focus of at least one diopter in magnitude showed a preference for grating orientation that was orthogonal to that focused myopically. When the infants were subsequently tested with optical correction, the preference for one orientation was no longer evident.

Thus, it appears that the defocus that is produced by astigmatism can have a measurable effect on the visual acuity of infants. This raises the issue of whether infantile astigmatism should be corrected. On the one hand, the data from Teller et al. (1978) and Held (1978) suggest that correction of the astigmatism can result in better acuity for infants. However, on the other hand, astigmatism in infants is very labile and in most infants it is gone by the time they reach 1 1/2 to 2 years of age (Held, 1978; Atkinson et al., 1980; Howland, 1982). This means that that any attempt to provide adequate correction for an infant's astigmatism would require frequent monitoring of the infant's refractive error. Further research on the long-term effects of uncorrected infantile astigmatism would help clinicians decide the extent to which optical correction would be beneficial to individual astigmatic infants.

Monocular vs. binocular testing. All of the normative acuity data shown in Figures 2 and 3 for infants and toddlers were obtained with binocular testing. However, it would be of much more value clinically to have data on normative acuity values obtained monocularly.

Atkinson et al. (1982) compared monocular vs. binocular acuity in 16 3- to 4- month old infants and found that there was a tendency for binocular acuity to be slightly better than monocular acuity, although the difference was less than one octave[3]. Atkinson et al. suggest that the distraction of wearing a patch during monocular testing may have contributed to the reduced monocular acuity shown by some of the infants.

Mayer et al. (1982) conducted monocular PL acuity testing in 16 infants who ranged in age from 2 months to 4 years. They compared their results with previously-obtained binocular acuity data and found, as did Atkinson et al. (1982), that monocular and binocular acuity values differed by less than one octave, but there was a tendency for the monocular values to be less than the binocular values.

[3]An octave is a halving or doubling of acuity, e.g., from 15 cy/deg to 30 cy/deg, or 20/40 to 20/20.

These studies suggest that, as a first approximation, normative acuity data obtained with binocular testing can be used as an indicator of whether a child's monocular acuity is within the normal range. Undoubtedly, within the next few years enough data will be published to allow the development of monocular PL acuity norms.

Acuity tasks. Acuity tasks can be divided into four types -- detection, recognition, resolution, and localization (Riggs, 1965). Clinical testing of adults typically measures recognition acuity, with either the Snellen letter chart or the Landolt C test. With infants and children, however, it is impossible to use these tests. Instead, researchers have concentrated on the development of procedures that measure resolution acuity, usually with black-and-white square- or sine-wave gratings.

One study, however, tested infants with stimuli similar to those used in studies of detection acuity in adults. Lewis et al (1978) compared the fixation times shown by 150 newborn infants for a homogeneous black field to their fixation times for single white lines of varying widths, presented on a black field. Their results showed that the newborns fixated a line 8 min. in width longer than they fixated the blank field, but there was no difference in duration of fixation for a 4 min. line as compared with a blank field. This acuity value of 8 min. is considerably better than the value of 20 min. that has been measured to be the resolution acuity of very young (2-week-old) infants (Fantz et al., 1962; Allen, 1979). Therefore, it appears that infants, like adults, show better acuity with detection stimuli than with resolution stimuli.

Stimulus eccentricity. The only researchers that have looked at acuity for stimuli at different eccentricities are Lewis et al (1978), in their study of acuity for single line stimuli. In that study, 150 newborn infants were shown single white lines of varying widths at 10, 20, and 30 degrees from a central fixation stimulus, and direction of first fixation was recorded for each infant's left eye. The results showed that the threshold line widths for stimuli presented on the subject' left (i.e., in the temporal field) were 33 min. for stimuli at 10 and 20 degrees, and 1 degree 6 min. for stimuli at 30 degrees. When the stimuli were presented on the right (i.e., in the nasal field) the threshold line width detected by the infants for stimuli at 10 degrees was 1 degree 6 min. For stimuli presented 20 and 30 degrees to the right, the infants showed no evidence that they detected any of the stimulus lines. These results suggest that stimulus eccentricity does affect visual acuity in infants and that, at least for newborn infants, acuity may be very different in the nasal vs. the temporal visual field.

Temporal properties of the stimulus. Researchers who have used the VEP to measure acuity in infants have typically found better acuity values than those obtained with PL procedures in infants of the same age (see Dobson and Teller, 1978b, for a review). It has been suggested (Dobson and Teller, 1978a; Sokol, 1978) that stimulus differences might account for at least some of the difference in acuity found between the two techniques, since VEP studies use temporally-modulated (phase-alternated or flashed) stimuli and PL studies typically use static gratings. Similarly, it might be suggested that use of a temporally-modulated stimulus in a PL procedure might improve acuity results by making the stimuli more salient or interesting to infants.

Two studies have compared acuity values for temporally-modulated vs. stationary stimuli in individual infants tested with the PL procedure. Atkinson et al. (1977b) measured 1- to 3-month-old infants' acuity and contrast sensitivity for drifting (3 Hz) vs. stationary sine-wave gratings. They found that although infants were more sensitive to moving gratings at low spatial frequencies, there was no difference in infants' acuity for moving vs. stationary gratings. Similarly, Dobson et al. (1978) found no difference in 2-month-old infants' acuity for stationary square-wave gratings vs. phase-alternated checkerboards similar to those often used in VEP studies. Thus, at least for the relatively restricted stimulus conditions and age range used by Atkinson et al., and Dobson et al., temporal modulation of acuity stimuli has no measureable effect on the acuity of young infants.

Gestational age. Finally, there is a factor that is of considerably more importance in studies of infants than in studies of adults. This factor is the gestational age of the subject at birth. One might hypothesize that infants born prior to term would show visual acuity development similar to that of full-term infants of the same postnatal age, since they have had the same amount of exposure to visual stimulation as the full-term infants. However, this does not occur; when preterm infants are compared to full-term infants of the same postnatal age, the visual acuity of preterm infants is consistently poorer than that of full-term infants (Fantz et al., 1965, Dobson et al., 1980). In fact, the visual acuity development of the preterm infant is much closer to that of full-term infants of the same post-conceptual age. Thus, if one is attempting to determine whether a preterm infant's acuity development is normal, the results obtained with the infant should be compared with the results of full-term infants who are the same age from conception (not the same age from birth) as the preterm infant.

In summary, there are a number of parameters that can affect visual acuity in both infants and adults. Although a few researchers have begun to look at these parameters in infants, most of the studies have been limited because only a few subjects in a very limited age range -- usually 2 to 4 months postnatal age -- were tested. Further exploration of these parameters should enhance the clinical utility of PL procedures.

IV. CLINICAL USEFULNESS OF PL PROCEDURES

To date, relatively few studies of the clinical usefulness of PL procedures have been published, and many of those that have been published are in the form of case reports. The following paragraphs give an indication of the types of eye disorders in which PL procedures have provided useful clinical information.

Strabismus. Several studies have used the PL procedure to estimate monocular acuities in infants with congenital esotropia (Thomas et al., 1979; Mohindra et al., 1980; Katsumi et al., 1981; Jacobson et al., 1982; Atkinson et al., 1982; Mayer, et al., 1982). These studies suggest that the PL procedure is helpful both in assessing the extent to which amblyopia is present and in monitoring the effect of occlusion therapy.

An example of the usefulness of PL procedures with strabismic infants can be seen in Figure 6. This figure plots data from a congenitally esotropic infant whose monocular PL acuity was followed for several months before and during occlusion therapy (Jacobson et al., 1982). When the child was first examined, at 19 weeks, clinical examination revealed a constant esotropia of the right eye of 45 prism diopters. At that time, acuity as measured with the PL procedure was equal in the two eyes. When the child's acuity was tested at 28 weeks, however, there was a large difference between eyes, with the acuity of the left eye being 2 octaves better than the acuity of the right eye. Occlusion therapy of the left eye for one hour per day was started when the infant was 30.5 weeks old. During the following four weeks, acuity in the right eye improved, while acuity in the left eye got worse. Occlusion was then changed to one hour per day, alternating day-by-day the eye that was occluded. During the next seven weeks there was little difference in acuity between eyes.

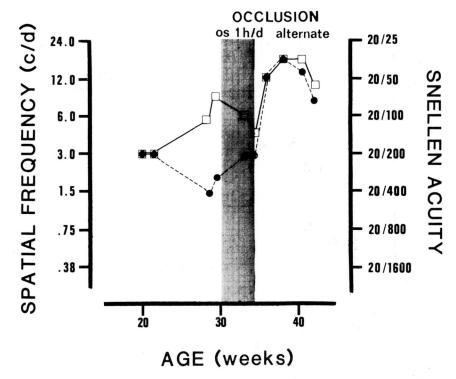

Figure 6. Visual acuity of an infant with congenital esotropia, as measured with preferential looking. At 20 and 22 weeks, acuity was much better in the non-deviating left eye than in the deviating right eye. Occlusion of the left eye for one hour per day was carried out from 30.5 to 34.5 weeks. During this time, acuity decreased in the non-deviating eye and improved in the deviating eye. Subsequently, occlusion was changed to one hour per day, with the alternate eye occluded on each day, and acuity remained approximately equal until the conclusion of testing, at 42 weeks. (Jacobson et al., 1982. Published with permission from The American Journal of Ophthamology Copyright by The Ophthamology Publishing Company.)

Anisometropia. PL procedures have also been used in the clinical assessment of visual acuity in infants and young children with anisometropia (Atkinson et al., 1982; Mayer et al., 1982). Mayer et al.'s results from 12 children with anisometropia who were tested before treatment are shown in Figure 7. The figure shows that before treatment, the acuity difference between eyes varied systematically with the amount of anisometropia present. Follow-up testing of four of these children showed that following optical correction, a significant reduction in the acuity difference between eyes was obtained for a 6-month-old with 1.5 diopters of anisometropia, a 22-month-old with 3.5 diopters of anisometropia, and a 4-year-old with 0.9 diopter of anisometropia. The fourth child, who was 5 years old

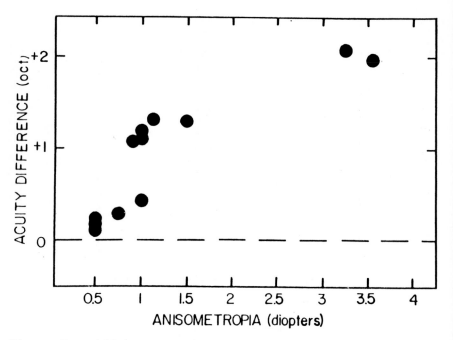

Figure 7. Differences between right eye and left eye acuities obtained with the OPL procedure, as a function of the amount of anisometropia. The subjects had no major ocular abnormalities and at least 0.5 diopter difference in spherical equivalent between eyes. Each point represents data from one child. The ordinate gives the difference, in octaves, between monocular acuities proportional to the better acuity, and the abscissa gives the difference between eyes in spherical equivalent. The acuity difference between eyes increased with increasing anisometropia. (Reprinted with permission from Mayer et al. 1982.)

at the time of optical correction, continued to show a significant acuity difference between eyes following optical correction and is currently undergoing occlusion therapy for amblyopia.

Suspected blindness. A recent case in our laboratory emphasized for us the usefulness of PL procedures as a supplement to the fixation and following procedures used by physicians to evaluate vision in very young infants. A two-month-old infant who was born 4 weeks prior to term was referred to us because he showed no evidence of vision; he would not fixate or follow any stimulus. In the PL procedure, however, his visual ability was clear; he showed a strong fixation preference for the striped targets and showed visual acuity results similar to those shown by normal one-month-olds. Subsequent testing at three and four months (two and three months from due date) showed that his acuity was normal when compared with that of infants of the same age from due date. Also, by three and four months, he was showing evidence of vision, as assessed by fixation and following. These results emphasize the point that PL procedures can provide a valuable addition to traditional methods of assessing vision in young infants.

Other ophthalmic abnormalities. PL procedures have also been used to assess visual acuity in infants and toddlers with a variety of other eye disorders, including congenital cataracts, ocular trauma, congenital nystagmus, ocular albinism, micropthalmia, coloboma, ptosis, optic nerve lesions, and retinal degeneration (see Atkinson et al., 1982; Jacobson, et al., 1982; Mayer et al., 1982).

Developmentally delayed children. A group of children who often have vision problems but who are very difficult to assess with standard clinical procedures are those children who are developmentally delayed. Mayer et al., (1981) used the OPL procedure to assess visual acuity in 69 children between the ages of 6 months and 16 years who were moderately to severely developmentally delayed. The group included children with seizure disorders, documented brain damage, severe cerebral palsy, and Downs' syndrome. Although only four of these children were testable with Allen picture cards, Mayer et al. were able to estimate acuity with the OPL procedure successfully in 61 of the 69 children (88%). Thus, PL procedures can be useful not only with infants and toddlers, but with older subjects who are developmentally immature.

V. SUMMARY AND CONCLUSIONS

In summary, PL techniques provide us with a behavioral measure of visual acuity that is more precise than other behavioral procedures that have been used to estimate acuity in non-verbal infants and young children. Preliminary studies suggest that PL procedures will be useful for clinical assessment of visual development as well as the laboratory investigation of the visual abilities of infants and young children. Nevertheless, some of the current limitations of PL procedures need to be considered and perhaps resolved before PL can become a widespread part of clinical practice.

1. One of the most notable limitations of all PL procedures is the lack of certainty of the acuity values obtained during the test. That is, because it is rarely possible to obtain a large number of trials with infants and toddlers, one's estimate of acuity is limited by the statistical variability inherent in a two-choice

situation (Banks et al., 1982; McKee et al., in preparation). Banks et al. (1982) and Mayer et al. (1982) have calculated that the PL procedures currently used for clinical estimation of visual acuity have a relatively large standard error of estimation and that acuity differences of less than one octave should not be considered reliable. Thus, if clinical PL testing revealed an acuity of 20/100 in one eye of a child and 20/50 in the other eye, one could be relatively confident that the acuity difference between eyes is real. However, a smaller acuity difference between eyes, for example, 20/30 vs. 20/50, might be due to the variability inherent in a PL procedure that employs a small number of trials. Furthermore, for infants younger than 6 months, Mayer et al. (1982) have calculated that differences of less than 1.5 octaves between eyes are not reliable.

2. A second limitation of PL procedures at the present time is the lack of normative data for children between 12 and 36 months of age. The PL procedures that have been developed for children in this age range are very new; therefore there has not yet been time for extensive normative data to be collected and to appear in print.

3. A third limitation of PL procedures, as far as any widespread clinical use, is that the procedures are evolving rapidly at the moment. The technique has only recently been introduced into clinical settings, and based on the early clinical results obtained in these settings, researchers have been modifying the procedure to attempt to make it quick and efficient in the clinic. The outcome of these initial clinical trials should define the settings in which the procedure will be most useful -- in specialized eye care centers as a supplemental tool for the assessment of diagnosed or suspected eye disorders, as a screening tool for early detection of visual problems, etc.

4. A fourth consideration, which may or may not be considered a limitation of the procedure by eye practitioners, is that PL procedures measure resolution acuity (acuity for a black-and-white grating), not recognition acuity (the acuity measured with a Snellen chart). Recent research has shown that there are ophthalmic conditions, most notably amblyopia, in which very different estimates of acuity are obtained with resolution than with recognition acuity tasks (Hess and Bradley, 1980; Levi and Klein, 1983). Thus, the PL acuity procedure may not provide the clinician with the information he or she would most like to have concerning amblyopic patients.

In conclusion, it is clear that PL techniques have provided researchers with a powerful tool for learning more about visual development in infants and young children. It is also clear that PL techniques can provide clinicians with knowledge about a non-verbal child's visual acuity development that cannot be obtained with any other currently-available behavioral assessment techniques. The extent to which the PL procedures will become a widespread clinical tool, however, depends to a large extent on the success with which researchers can improve on the above-mentioned limitations and the extent to which a procedure that retains some of these limitations can provide helpful information to the clinician.

Supported by NIH grant EY 02581.

REFERENCES

Allen, J. 1979. Visual acuity development in human infants up to 6 months of age. Unpublished doctoral dissertation, University of Washington.

Atkinson, J. 1977. Contrast sensitivity in the infant. In Spatial Contrast. Edited by H. Spekreijse and L.D. van der Tweel. North Holland, Amsterdam.

Atkinson, J. and O. Braddick. 1979. New techniques for assessing vision in infants and young children. Child: care, health and development 5; 389-398.

Atkinson, J., O. Braddick and J. French. 1980. Infant astigmatism: Its disappearance with age. Vis. Res. 20; 891-893.

Atkinson, J., O. Braddick and K. Moar. 1977a. Development of contrast sensitivity over the first 3 months of life in the human infant. Vis. Res. 17; 1037-1044.

Atkinson, J., O. Braddick and K. Moar. 1977b. Contrast sensitivity of the human infant for moving and static patterns. Vis. Res. 17; 1045-1047.

Atkinson, J., O. Braddick and E. Pimm-Smith. 1982. 'Preferential looking' for monocular and binocular acuity testing of infants. Br. J. Ophthal. 66; 264-268.

Atkinson, J., J. French and O. Braddick. 1981. Contrast sensitivity function of preschool children. Br. J. Ophthal. 65; 525-529.

Banks, M.S. and P. Salapatek. 1976. Contrast sensitivity function of the infant visual system. Vis. Res. 16; 867-869.

Banks, M.S. and P. Salapatek. 1978. Acuity and contrast sensitivity of one-, two-, and three-month-old human infants. Invest. Ophthal. Vis. Sci. 17; 361-365.

Banks, M.S., B.R. Stephens and J.L. Dannemiller. 1982. A failure to observe negative preference in infant acuity testing. Vis. Res. 22; 1025-1031.

Berlyne, D.E. 1958. The influence of the albedo and complexity of stimuli on visual fixation in the human infant. Brit. J. Psychol. 49; 315-318.

Birch, E.E., J. Naegele, J.A. Bauer and R. Held. 1982. Visual acuity of toddlers tested by operant and preferential looking techniques. Paper presented at The Association for Research in Vision and Ophthalmology Spring Meeting, Orlando, Florida, May 4-9, 1980.

Campbell, F.W. 1957. The depth of field of the human eye. Optica Acta 4; 157-164.

Committee on Vision. 1980. Recommended Standard Procedures for the Clinical Measurement and Specification of Visual Acuity. Adv. Ophthal. 41; 103-148.

Dobson, V. 1980. Behavioral tests of visual acuity in infants. International Ophthalmology Clinics. Electrophysiology and Psychophysics. Their Use in Ophthalmic Diagnosis 20; 233-250.

Dobson, V., D.L. Mayer and C.P. Lee. 1980. Visual acuity screening of preterm infants. Invest. Ophthal. Vis. Sci. 19; 1498-1505.

Dobson, V., D. Salem and J.B. Carson. 1983. Visual acuity in infants: The effect of variations in stimulus luminance within the photopic range. Invest. Ophthal. Vis. Sci. 24:519-522.

Dobson, V. and D.Y. Teller. 1978. Assessment of visual acuity in infants. In: Visual Psychophysics and Physiology. Edited by J. Armington, J. Krauskopf and B. Wooten. Academic Press, New York.

Dobson, V. and D.Y. Teller. 1978. Visual acuity in human infants: A review and comparison of behavioral and electrophysiological studies. Vis. Res. 18; 1469-1483.

Dobson, V., D.Y. Teller and J. Belgum. 1978. Visual acuity in human infants assessed with stationary stripes and alternating checkerboards. Vis. Res. 18; 1233-1238.

Fantz, R.L. 1958. Pattern vision in young infants. Psychol. Rec. 8; 43-47.

Fantz, R.L., J.F. Fagan, III and S.B. Miranda. 1975. Early visual selectivity. In: Infant Perception: From Sensation to Cognition. Vol. 1. Basic Visual Processes. Edited by L.B. Cohen and P. Salapatek. Academic Press, New York.

Fantz, R.L., J. Ordy and M. Udelf. 1962. Maturation of pattern vision in infants during the first six months of life. J. Comp. Physiol. Psychol. 55; 907-917.

Fiorentini, A., M. Pirchio and D. Spinelli. 1980. Scotopic contrast sensitivity in infants evaluated by evoked potentials. Invest. Ophthal. Vis. Sci. 19; 950-955.

Fulton, A.B., V. Dobson, D. Salem, C. Mar, R. Petersen and R. Hansen. 1980. Cycloplegic refractions in infants and young children. Am. J. Ophthal. 90; 239-247.

Green, D.G., M.K. Powers and M.S. Banks. 1980. Depth of focus, eye size and visual acuity. Vis. Res. 20; 827-835.

Gstalder, R.J. and D.G. Green. 1971. Laser interferometric acuity in amblyopia. J. Ped. Ophthal. 8; 251-256.

Gwiazda, J., E. Birch and R. Held. 1981. Le developpement de la vision chez l'enfant. La Recherche 12; 1349-1353.

Gwiazda, J., S. Brill, I. Mohindra and R. Held. 1978. Infant visual acuity and its meridional variation. Vis. Res. 18; 1557-1564.

Gwiazda, J., S. Brill, I. Mohindra and R. Held. 1980. Preferential looking acuity in infants from two to fifty-eight weeks of age. Amer. J. Optom. Physiol. Opt. 57; 428-432.

Held, R. 1978. Development of visual acuity in normal and astigmatic infants. In Frontiers in Visual Science. Edited by S.J. Cool and E.L. Smith, III. Springer-Verlag, New York.

Held, R., I Mohindra, J. Gwiazda and S. Brill. 1977. Visual acuity of astigmatic infants and its meridional variation. Paper presented at The Association for Research in Vision and Ophthalmology Spring Meeting, Sarasota, Florida, April 25-29, 1977.

Hess, R.F. and Bradley, A. 1980. Contrast preception above threshold is only minimally impaired in human amblyopia. Nature. 287; 463-464.

Howland, H.C. 1982. Infant eyes: Optics and accommodation. Current Eye Research 2; 217-224.

Howland, H.C., J. Atkinson, O. Braddick and J. French. 1978. Infant astigmatism measured by photorefraction. Science 202; 331-333.

Ingram, R.M. and A. Barr. 1979. Changes in refraction between the ages of 1 and 3 1/2 years. Br. J. Ophthal. 63; 339–342.

Jacobson, S.G., I. Mohindra and R. Held. 1982. Visual acuity of infants with ocular diseases. Amer. J. Ophthal. 93; 198–209.

Katsumi, O., Y. Oguchi and Y. Uemura. 1981. Assessment of visual ability in infantile esotropia using preferential looking method. Jap. J. Ophthal. 25; 457–463.

Levi, D.N. and S. Klein. 1982. Differences in vernier discrimination for gratings between strabismic and anisometric amblyopes. Invest. Ophthal. Vis. Sci. 23: 398–407.

Lewis, T.L., D. Maurer and D. Kay. 1978. Newborns' central vision: Whole or hole? J. Exp. Child Psychol. 26; 193–203.

Lippmann, O. 1971. Vision screening of young children. Am. J. Publ. Health 61; 1586–1601.

Mayer, D.L. and V. Dobson. 1980. Assessment of vision in young children: A new operant approach yields estimates of acuity. Invest. Ophthal. Vis. Sci. 19; 566–570.

Mayer, D.L. and V. Dobson. 1982. Visual acuity development in infants and young children as assessed by operant preferential looking. Vis. Res. 22; 1141–1151.

Mayer, D.L., A.B. Fulton and R.M. Hansen. 1981. Visual acuity assessment of developmentally delayed infants and children using operant preferential looking (OPL). Paper presented at Biennial Meeting of Society for Research in Child Development, Boston, MA, April 3, 1981.

Mayer, D.L., A.B. Fulton and R.M. Hansen. 1982. Preferential looking acuity in pediatric patients obtained with a staircase procedure. Invest. Ophthal. Vis. Sci. 23; 538–543.

McKee, S., D. Teller and S. Klein. Statistical properties of forced-choice psychometric functions: Implications of probit analysis. In preparation.

Mohindra, I., R. Held, J. Gwiazda and S. Brill. 1978. Astigmatism in infants. Science 202; 329–331.

Mohindra, I., S.G. Jacobson, J. Thomas and R. Held. 1980. Development of amblyopia in infants. Trans. Ophthal. Soc. U. K. 99; 344–346.

Powers, M.K. and V. Dobson. 1982. Effect of focus on visual acuity of human infants. Vis. Res. 22; 521–528.

Riggs, L.A. 1965. Visual acuity. In: Vision and Visual Perception. Edited by C.H. Graham. Wiley & Sons, New York.

Roberts, J. and J. Ludford. 1977. Monocular visual acuity of persons 4-74 years. Vital Health Stats. Series 11; 1–31.

Salapatek, P., A.G. Bechtold and E.W. Bushnell. 1976. Infant visual acuity as a function of viewing distance. Child Develop. 47; 860–863.

Santonastaso, A. 1930. La rifrazione oculare nei primi anni di vita. Annali di ottalmologia e clinica oculista 58; 852–885.

Shlaer, S. 1937. The relation between visual acuity and illumination. J. Gen. Physiol. 21; 165–188.

Sokol, S. 1978. Measurement of infant visual acuity from pattern reversal evoked potentials. Vis. Res. 18; 33–39.

Teller, D.Y. 1979. The forced-choice preferential looking procedure: A psychophysical technique for use with human infants. Infant Behavior and Development 2; 135–153.

Teller, D.Y., J.L. Allen, D.M. Regal and D.L. Mayer. 1978. Astigmatism and acuity in two primate infants. Invest. Ophthal. Vis. Sci. 17:344–349.

Teller, D.Y., R. Morse, R. Borton and D. Regal. 1974. Visual acuity for vertical and diagonal gratings in human infants. Vis. Res. 14; 1433–1439.

Thomas, J., I. Mohindra and R. Held. 1979. Strabismic amblyopia in infants. Amer. J. Optom. Physiol. Opt. 56; 197–201.

Woodruff, M.E. 1972. Observations on the visual acuity of children during the first five years of life. Am. J. Optom. Arch. Am. Acad. Optom. 49; 205-215.

Discussion of the Papers by Drs. Sokol and Dobson

L. Riggs

Drs. Sokol and Dobson have given us clear accounts of the state of the art of evaluating visual sensitivity in young children. Each of them is to be congratulated on a broad coverage of the principal facts, together with a fair evaluation of both the advantages and the limitations of the methods they have discussed.

Dr. Sokol first shows the wide applicability of recording visually evoked cortical potentials (which I prefer to abbreviate as VECP) in the study of the developing visual system from birth to early childhood. But he is immediately confronted with the fact that the VECP seriously overestimates the acuity of infants as judged by behavioral methods. This fact is so puzzling as to cause him to obtain both VECP measures and behavioral ones based on a preferential looking (PL) technique with the same infants and with identical stimulus conditions. The discrepancy still shows up, however, and possible reasons for it must be considered. Dr. Sokol notes, for example, that Teller (1979) cautions that an infant may possibly be able to discriminate between a patterned and an unpatterned stimulus, yet not show a preference for the patterned one until its contours reach suprathreshold intensity. That possibility must indeed be kept in mind for all psychophysical studies based upon preference rather than discrimination. The two-bottle taste preference studies of animals have long been under suspicion as valid determiners of taste thresholds.

In his summary, Dr. Sokol points out a possible weakness of VECP recording as a measure of vision: The potentials arise mainly from the occipital cortex and do not reflect possible further processing that may underlie subjective visual experience. This, too, is a valid argument. In my own laboratory VECP signals have failed to be diminished under conditions in which the subject reports the disappearance of the eliciting stimulus due to binocular rivalry or due to stabilization of the retinal image.

In all these VECP studies, computer averaging techniques have necessarily been employed. As Dr. Sokol points out, this may conceivably cause subthreshold signals to emerge above the ambient noise. This point deserves particular emphasis. To put it another way, the integration time of the human visual system is in the range of tenths of a second, whereas computer averaging involves integration over many seconds or even minutes of time. Thus the computer, rather than the brain may furnish the relatively noise-free signal that slowly emerges as the subject is marginally able, or sometimes unable, to see the eliciting stimulus pattern.

Despite the above reservations in regard to use of the VECP, one must admit that it has great potential usefulness for clinical diagnosis of individual cases, as Dr. Sokol has shown. Certain compromises have been made, no doubt, to simplify and speed up the recording that must be done, sometimes under difficulties such as limited time available for testing with an uncooperative subject. One could wish that the test stimulus could always be a sinusoidal grating of variable contrast and variable spatial frequency. That would permit the derivation, for each eye tested, of a complete contrast sensitivity function such as that used in the most advanced of our clinical laboratories. But this would require much more time, and the signals would typically be weak compared to those shown in this paper for square-wave grating or checkerboard patterns of stimulation. The complexity of these patterns should be kept in mind, however, in interpreting the "spatial frequency" results in Figures 2 and 3, since the abscissa does not indicate the higher harmonics that are also present in each stimulus.

Even more complex is the matter of using negative spherical lenses to evaluate accommodation. It is a fact that there is much less loss of contrast in the retinal image of a poorly accommodated coarse target than in that of a fine target. Thus one must carefully distinguish the effects of faulty accommodation from those of spatial frequency in causing blur and the attendant reduction of VECP signal strength. With regard to Figure 7, for example, statements in the text may be questioned. Specifically, the apparently more successful accommodation with large check sizes may result instead from less blur and a loss of contrast for large checks as compared to small ones even when accommodation is off by the same amount for both. This question could be cleared up if an independent measure of accommodation (such as that of Haynes et al., 1965) were available.

Dr. Sokol has shown that, despite necessary compromises of methodology and interpretation, the VECP technique is of proven usefulness in the study of early visual development.

Dr. Dobson starts off with an account of how psychophysical data have been obtained on visual sensitivity in human infants. The basic technique, as in earlier studies with experimental anaimals, is to take advantage of a naturally occurring behavioral response to the stimulus. But instead of using a primitive reflex, such as optokinetic nystagmus or an orienting response, the trick is to measure the extent to which an infant prefers to look at a test pattern rather than a blank field. The underlying assumption is that any pattern the infant can see will attract earlier and more frequent fixations than a field in which no pattern is visible. As we have noted above, this assumption raises questions about how far above the threshold of discrimination a pattern must be in order to induce the preferential looking. But the original observations of Berlyne and Fantz have been supported by elegant psychophysical experiments of Teller and her colleagues, showing that highly reliable developmental data are obtained by this technique. We can perhaps console ourselves with the thought that what matters is not to measure the lowest possible threshold of discrimination but rather to arrive at any index of visual function that can usefully be applied in comparative studies of the effects of age or of clinical or experimental conditions. As Dr. Dobson has shown us, the forced choice preferential looking technique has served as such an index with particular success up to the age of six months. And it is significant that various reinforcement procedures extend its usefulness for older children. Is it too wild an idea that rein- forcement could work for those younger than six months as well? Cheerios, no! But maybe milk or mush? The use of reinforcement at all ages might have the advantage of better comparability in the developmental studies, and a greater probability that threshold levels of discrimination would be manifested by the data.

Dr. Dobson, like Dr. Sokol, has made use of strong lenses to defocus the optical image. Again the matter is complex, and data such as those in Fig. 5 must be viewed with caution. Any human subject, or any camera, will show greater effects of defocus on high spatial frequency images than on low. That fact is just as true an interpretation of Fig. 5 as the one given, namely that adults suffer a greater loss of acuity than do infants wearing lenses of the same power. If it were possible to obtain a full contrast sensitivity function for an infant, one might find that the sensitivity was no worse, and perhaps even better, than that of an adult in the region of low spatial frequencies. By the same token, an infant might suffer as great a loss as would an adult when the same coarse gratings were viewed by each through defocussing lenses.

Dr. Dobson is right in advocating the use of gestational age rather than age since birth in developmental studies. A logarithmic scaling of gestational age may then be appropriate for expressing developmental data. But the logarithmic scaling of age since birth (see Fig. 8) should certainly be avoided. Such a scale would imply that there is as much development from the first hour to the tenth hour after birth as there is from the first month to the tenth!

All in all, Dr. Dobson has made a good case for using behavioral tests in studies of visual development. This is especially true when proper forced-choice procedures are carried out by observers who are judging the infant's direction of regard without being allowed to see the true location of the stimulus, and when adequate numbers of trials are given for statistical reliability. We may confidently expect further significant improvement in this relatively new means of evaluating developmental, clinical and experimental determiners of visual function.

Index